More Medicode Products: Coder-Tested And Coder-Approved

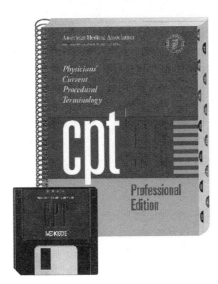

Color Keys And Illustrations For 1996

Using updated codes is essential. That's why *CPT 1996* is a must for every office. Easy to use, *CPT 1996* is the most comprehensive coding reference available for CPT codes.

New CPT 1996 Professional Edition

The AMA's new *Professional Edition of CPT 1996* delivers the features of the standard edition, plus:

- **Color Keys.** These easy-to-see keys support precision coding.

- **Anatomical Illustrations.** They make coding more manageable.

- **Medical Terminology.** Defines and clarifies complex meanings.

- **Spiral Binding And Thumb-Index Tabs.** Facilitate handling and use.

CPT On Disk

With *Medicode's Relative Values And CPT 1996 On Disk* you'll get CPT codes, abbreviated descriptions and Medicode's relative values. DOS ASCII file imports easily into your software.

New Color-Coding For Ease-Of-Use

You'll need our *HCPCS 1996* to bill Medicare and many private payers. It's the most user-friendly, most comprehensive edition on the market. And new features for this year:

- New color coding of Medicare coverage instructions with a helpful legend.

- Expanded index that includes product name references. Find products, even if you don't know the manufacturer.

- Thinner size and free spiral binding.

Plus these existing features:

- Pharmacist-verified table of drugs with brand names, generics, dosage, route of administration and correct J or K codes.

- Instructions preceding each section to guide you through information.

HCPCS On Disk

With *HCPCS 1996 On Disk* you'll get HCPCS Level II codes and full descriptions. DOS ASCII file imports easily into your software.

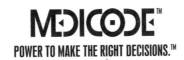

MEDICODE™

POWER TO MAKE THE RIGHT DECISIONS.™

Available from your medical bookstore or distributor. For a free catalog, call 1-800-999-4600.

More Medicode Products:
Coder-Tested And Coder-Approved

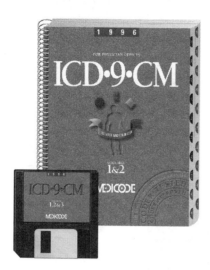

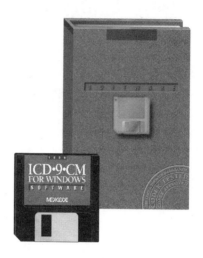

Coding With An Outdated ICD-9 Is Risky

Not a single *Medicode ICD•9* goes out until every one of the government's code changes are included. So only Medicode dares to offer this risk-free guarantee: "Use any *Medicode 1996 ICD•9*. If you make a coding error based on an outdated code, Medicode will give you next year's *ICD•9* absolutely free!" But that's not all.

Receive Our New Specialty Minibook FREE!

Order a *Deluxe 1996 ICD•9* and get our handy new *ICD•9 Minibook,* free. It organizes codes by specialty (eight in all). Plus, our *Deluxe ICD•9* includes quality spiral binding and thumb-index tabs.

Minibook Specialties Available:

Cardiology • General Surgery • Primary Care • Ophthalmology • Obstetrics And Gynecology • OMS And Reconstructive Surgery • Orthopedics • Urology

New for 1996, our *Compact ICD•9* is easier to handle, at just 6" x 9" and with thumb-index tabs. It includes the same features as our *Standard 1996 ICD•9*, but takes up less space on your desk.

Our ICD-9 Software Opens New Windows

Medicode's new *ICD•9 For Windows* gives you most everything that's in our printed *ICD•9*, plus the ease-of-use and added features of software.

- Displays tabular and index information.

- Uses Medicode's exclusive color coding system.

- Contains all tabular ICD•9 codes in *Volumes 1 & 3*, and uses all terms from the *Volume 2* index in its searching capability.

- Includes complete long descriptions, includes, excludes, notes and "Use additional ..." instructions.

- Lets you search by code or description and save your search criteria for future use.

- Instantly prints reports.

- Displays pop-up warnings for codes requiring additional digits, non-specific codes and secondary diagnoses.

- Lets you paste codes and descriptions into your billing software and other documents.

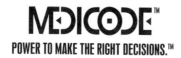

POWER TO MAKE THE RIGHT DECISIONS.™

PATIENT CONFIDENTIALITY

AN ALPHABETIZED GUIDE TO THE RELEASE OF MEDICAL INFORMATION

By Janet M. McGee, R.R.A.

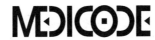

ISBN 1-56337-122-7

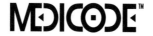

Medicode, Inc.
5225 Wiley Post Way, Suite 500
Salt Lake City, UT 84116-2889

Medicode Publishing Staff

Publisher	Susan P. Seare
Editorial Director	Lynn Speirs
Medical Director	Jerry G. Seare, M.D.
Project Editor	Robert J. Welsh
Research Editor	Tricia Phillips
Layout	Cheryl S. Bosh

Acknowledgements

Grateful acknowledgement is made to: Medicode and the company's publisher, Susan Seare, for their show of faith; my editor Bob Welsh, for his patience, good humor, and hard work; Tricia Phillips for the very thorough research that constitutes appendix 1; Anne Wangman, R.R.A., and Marcia Loellbach of the American Health Information Management Association for their wonderfully efficient help in researching information, tracking down individuals, and quick turnarounds on permission granted to use material published in the Association's journal; Helen Marek, R.R.A., for permission to incorporate material from her *Medicolegal Guidelines and Forms for Hospitals* and, more importantly her encouragement in the early stages of the project; Kim Roeder of the law firm Powell, Goldstein, Frazer and Murphy in Atlanta for granting permission to use material from H. Boyce Connell, Jr.'s *Georgia Law of Medical Records;* Carmen Petrin, R.N., of the New Hampshire Nurses' Association's Commission on Continuing Education for her help and encouragement in preparing the application for approval of the continuing education module for the American Nurses' Association; Lorraine Gordon, R.N., Yvette Raleigh, R.N.C., and Anita Thomas, R.N.C., of the Portsmouth (NH) Regional Hospital for serving as members of the planning committee for the Independent Study and Seminar Programs and for their help with the pilot program; Darryl Lundeen, R.N.C., Diane Geraci, L.P.N., and Judy Downing, R.N.C., also of the Portsmouth (NH) Regional Hospital for the help with the pilot for the Independent Study Program; and my mom, Louise McGee, for her unwavering support of this project.

My heartfelt thanks to Bonnie A. Newton, R.R.A., a training specialist with the Columbia, Md., Medical Plan, for her unfailing friendship, professional counsel, and editing prowess.

About the Author   **Janet M. McGee**

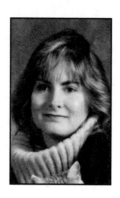

Experience

Ms. McGee is a Registered Record Administrator (R.R.A.) affiliated with the American Health Information Management Association. She also is a member of the American Veterinary Health Information Management Association.

Ms. McGee holds a B.S. Degree in Medical Record Administration, and is a graduate of the Health Record Administration Program, U.S. Public Health Service Hospital in Baltimore.

Ms. McGee is a businesswoman and independent health care management consultant, specializing in health insurance, risk management, and physician practice management. She has served as health records administrator and quality control manager for CompuHealth and has worked as a claims specialist for Blue Cross/Blue Shield, both of Atlanta. Additionally, she has served as chief financial counselor and CHAMPUS health benefits advisor for the Wyman Park Health System (formerly the U.S. Public Health Service Hospital) in Baltimore. She has also acted as supervisor for outpatient billing and liaison to ambulatory care at the U.S. Public Health Service Hospital.

Table of Contents

Foreword

Professional liability claims against healthcare providers and facilities have increased significantly during recent years. Both the number of claims and the average payment per claim settled has increased. Effective risk management practices can help minimize the adverse effects of these claims upon the healthcare provider.

Claims against healthcare providers frequently fall within an identifiable pattern. By identifying problem areas encountered in practice, risk management guidelines can be established to help prevent claims from arising. Claims against healthcare providers are frequently generated in the following areas:

▶ Referrals

▶ Adverse and/or unexpected results from medical treatment

▶ Lack of informed consent

▶ Inadequate record keeping

▶ Abandonment

▶ Breach of confidentiality/security of medical information

▶ Deficiencies in interaction between healthcare providers, staff, and patients.

This book should prove to be especially helpful on the above areas of confidentiality, security, and recordkeeping.

Professional liability insurance helps reduce the financial consequences of a substantial professional liability claim that could severely impact the healthcare provider. And, although such insurance can be a "safety net" for catastrophic losses, you can do a great deal to prevent claims from arising. Better communication with patients, improved record keeping and security techniques, clear and effective chart documentation, organized and well-considered treatment plans, and the preservation of well-documented (and unaltered) records can help reduce the chances of embarrassing and costly litigation.

In addition, attention to risk management can improve patient care while at the same time relieving the anxiety often felt by healthcare providers in today's difficult medical/legal climate. It is a delicate art to balance efficient use of auxiliary staff and treatment for cost efficiency with the need for the patients to feel that the healthcare provider cares and is involved adequately in the treatment process.

Understanding and Preventing Liability Claims

Professional liability claims often result from the unrealistic expectations of patients, bad results from treatment, and poor communication between the healthcare provider and the patient. And, in the area of confidentiality, the unauthorized release of medical information by uninformed or poorly trained personnel is very frequently problematic. A healthcare provider is generally defined as a person, partnership, association, corporation, or other facility or institution that renders, or causes to be rendered, healthcare or professional services. This includes but is not limited to hospitals, clinics, private physician practices, or nurses or agents of any of the above acting in the course and scope of their employment.

Malpractice is in essence a form of negligence, which is usually defined as (1) the failure to do something that a reasonable and prudent man, guided by those ordinary considerations that ordinarily regulate human affairs, would do, or (2) doing something that a reasonable and prudent man would not do. Negligence is based upon the breach of a duty on the part of one person to exercise care to protect another against injury. Negligence is a failure to observe a legal duty.

Vicarious Liability — Respondeat Superior

Even though a healthcare provider such as a physician may not have personally been negligent, he or she may bear liability exposure for the wrongful acts of others employed by them. This is referred to as "vicarious liability" or respondeat superior (literally, "let the master pay"), and is based upon the principle that the "master" should pay or be held responsible for the wrongful acts of the people who work for or are under his or her control and supervision. Thus, the most careful physician can face significant liability exposure for improperly trained staff. Since physicians seldom personally handle such routine matters as responding to requests for information and the general security of the medical records, they should conduct an efficient risk management overview of the entire office in an effort to correct any perceived deficiencies or problem areas.

Health Histories

One of the most important elements in a patient's complete medical record is the health history. Healthcare providers are well advised to record and maintain a proper medical history for each patient. Many claims against healthcare providers can be avoided if adequate medical histories are taken to assist in the diagnosis or treatment.

Many forms are available for recording a patient's medical history, and this is one area where the auxiliary staff can efficiently assist the healthcare provider. The office staff should be involved in having patients fill-out these forms and in supplementing and updating them at regular treatment intervals. These health histories should be consistently completed, dated, and signed by the patient, and the forms can be tailored to the specific needs and specialty of your practice.

Include in these health histories any health problems that may enter into the evaluation of the risks involved in any contemplated medical procedure or treatment plan. The completed health history alerts you to any health hazards the patient may present and to possible negative effects a treatment may produce in a given patient. Discuss the completed health history form with the patient prior to the start of any procedure. Responses that lead you to suspect that a patient is presenting symptoms that reflect underlying medical problems will prompt additional questioning. As a rule, do not delegate the review of the form and discussion with the patient to a staff member.

Record Keeping and Release of Records

Keep a separate medical record file for each patient. This file should contain (1) the patient's health history and updates, (2) copies of any signed consent forms or contemporaneous entries documenting the discussion regarding informed consent with the patient, (3) the results of laboratory studies and x-ray interpretations, (4) copies of all prescriptions and clear documentation of medications being taken by patients, (5) a treatment summary for each office visit, (6) a summary of telephone conversations with the patient, (7) scheduled appointments and missed appointments, (8) referral notations or consultations concerning other healthcare providers and consent to release information forms. Standardize all your abbreviations.

The SOAP charting method is extremely helpful for standardizing and segmenting office visits. Briefly, the physician would record and structure an encounter as follows:

S = subjective	Patient's complaints, symptoms, etc.
O = objective	Physical data (exam, lab results, etc.)
A = assessment	Address each problem or diagnosis separately
P = plan	List separately for each problem or diagnosis

Keep the records for a long period of time; statutes of limitations differ between states and jurisdictions. In particular, many claims involving minors are tolled until after the minor reaches majority, meaning that many stale claims can be brought years after the healthcare was rendered. Long term record retention is necessary.

Records should not be altered or changed at any time after a lawsuit is filed. Defense lawyers would much rather defend on an incomplete or absent record than on one that has been fraudulently altered. Handwriting experts are frequently retained to review cases for late entries or for entries that have been altered, and many cases that may otherwise be defensible may be lost due to a fraudulent change of records.

Do not correct errors by using "White Out" corrective fluid or by erasing. It is best to draw a single line through the incorrect entry so that it is still legible, then write the correct entry into the record above it. Sign and date the change and indicate why it was made. Make all comments in the record brief and to the point, avoiding inappropriate comments because of the prejudice created if the record must be later produced.

If a patient is involved in litigation, the proper preservation of the medical chart, laboratory studies and/or radiographs, and billing ledgers is essential. Most hospitals handle patient charts in litigation in a special manner by placing them in a different location under lock and key for protection and preservation. This practice can also be helpful in an office or clinic setting.

If a professional liability claim is filed against a healthcare provider, keep correspondence with the insurance carrier and with the defense attorney in a separate location from the treatment record. These materials are afforded certain protections under law from disclosure and should not be readily volunteered as part of the patient's treatment record being released.

Release of Medical Records

The issue of who owns the medical record (the healthcare provider or the patient) has been debated for decades. It is generally recognized that a healthcare provider has the right to maintain and preserve the original treatment record, but that the patient has a right of access to the record upon appropriate request. Because of the physician/patient privilege, it is important to maintain confidentiality concerning the patient's treatment and records reflecting that treatment.

Obtain a written authorization (required in many states) for medical release from a patient before releasing records to third parties. In the case of minors, a parent or the legal guardian, and in the case of a deceased patient, the personal representative or an heir should provide authorization before those records are released to third persons.

It is best not to release original x-rays and records in the absence of a subpoena or court order — even then the healthcare provider may want to consult with counsel before complying.

There is a lazy practice among some attorneys to attempt to obtain medical records across state lines without a patient release by use of an out-of-state subpoena. A subpoena from one state requesting records in another state is not valid unless that subpoena has been properly issued and authorized by the state wherein it is served. Be extra cautious before responding to an out-of-state subpoena (as opposed to a signed and notarized medical release) before producing records.

Conclusion

The best way to avoid a professional liability claim is, of course, to provide quality healthcare. However, this is not exclusively the cause of much litigation. For physicians, a better understanding of the medical/legal climate, attention to problematic areas within their practices, a competent and well-trained staff, and becoming aware of the problems outlined in this book will go a long way toward making your practice of the art and science of medicine more enjoyable and trouble free.

May 1993

David H. Epperson, Attorney at Law

(Mr. Epperson, of Hanson, Epperson & Smith in Salt Lake City, specializes in medical malpractice litigation/professional liability defense.)

Introduction

This guide is an alphabetized presentation of the numerous factors relating to the release of medical information. The body of the guide is preceded by an alphabetical Index. Key-word indexing and cross-referencing provide a thorough directory to the book, and you are encouraged to peruse this index when searching for information — it will save you considerable time when looking up items.

The material presented under each topic heading highlights in a brief, concise manner the major and prevailing principles, procedures, and issues regarding the release of medical information. Respective state statutes, federal law, and established facility or provider policies must always take precedence when referring to this "generic" guide.

This book has been formatted with a notational column next to the entries for two reasons. Firstly, students are encouraged to use this guide as a training tool; there is ample room for making notes relating to a topic referenced on a given page. Secondly, and ideally, the book can be customized in the space provided so that it reflects your specific state statutes and established employer policies.

My objectives in preparing this guide were threefold: (1) to provide a quick and easy-to-use reference to issues relating to the release of medical information, (2) to aid individuals involved in handling requests for information in achieving a comfort zone and confidence regarding any request (or demand) that comes their way, and (3) to promote the protection of a patient's right to privacy as well as the interests of the facility or provider releasing the information.

Medical Records and Confidentiality

A medical record is created and maintained for the benefit of the patient, the physician, and/or the treating healthcare facility. Although the physical record is the property of the provider, the information contained therein belongs to the patient.

Physicians, by virtue of having taken the Hippocratic Oath, have historically been charged with the responsibility of keeping patients' medical information confidential. However, the actual day-to-day burden of responding to requests for information usually falls upon the shoulders of a facility's or physician's employees.

A request for medical information is usually initiated in one of three ways:

- ▶ A formal request is made pursuant to a requirement such as a state statute, federal law, or regulation, often taking the form of a subpoena or court order.

- ▶ An informal request is made by the patient or other third party having need of the information.

- ▶ Information is voluntarily (e.g., juvenile drug use) or involuntarily (e.g., child abuse) reported by individuals having knowledge of certain situations. Voluntary disclosures are regulated by permissive disclosure laws that allow but do not require the disclosure of information.

When deciding what response should be made to a request for information, the most important elements to consider are the identity and authority of any party making a request, and the nature of the record and the information contained within. Currently, those areas generally considered to be especially sensitive and problematic with regard to releasing information are psychiatric (mental health) treatment, AIDS/HIV treatment, drug and/or alcohol abuse treatment records, and treatment of minors for certain conditions.

Generally, when analyzing laws and trying to determine which ones apply and should take precedence with regard to a specific issue, the strictest law applies. But, laws should only be considered the minimum standard. When developing a policy, you would do well to be even stricter than the law in your protection of the patient and his or her medical information. When this is done, however, be sure to indicate clearly in your policy statement the difference between what is required by law and your policy.

The recent emphasis on outpatient care has caused much of the "action" to move away from hospitals or acute care settings. As a result, too few of those responsible for the release of medical information are knowledgeable about the issues relating to it, specifically the major principles and generally accepted procedures and the ramifications of failing to abide by them. This knowledge shortage stems from a lack of traditional in-service training by health record professionals and/or a facility's legal counsel, and the lack of any quick and easy comprehensive guide. In addition, the increased use of personal computers to store medical information and the ever-increasing volume of requests and uses of information have contributed to an almost laissez-faire attitude toward an issue which, paradoxically, has such potential for unwanted legal action.

Managing Risks in Your Practice

Anytime an employee of a facility or physician endangers a patient's right to confidentiality — especially with an adverse or harmful outcome — that employee can be held liable. Physicians and/or facility administrators need to know that a finding for punitive damages on behalf of a plaintiff for mistakes made in releasing the plaintiff's medical information can severely affect their financial well-being. In many states punitive damages, designed to punish the facility or person responsible, are not insurable. They are uninsured losses, the amount of which will be based on the physician's or facility's net worth — a very unhappy circumstance. You are well advised to know the law and philosophy of your respective state and the policy of your malpractice carrier with regard to punitive damages and negligence in releasing medical information. Usually, one of three possibilities applies: (1) a state law does not allow for levying punitive damages, (2) punitive damages are allowed, but malpractice carriers do not automatically insure for them, or (3) punitive damages are allowed and are usually automatically provided for in policies underwritten by malpractice carriers.

The practices set forth here are those found to be generally consistent among all resources consulted. This guide is in no way a substitute for legal counsel and/or a working knowledge of laws and policies relevant to your particular situation. This generic guide, presenting generally accepted practices adaptable to multiple types of facilities or healthcare providers, is a good first reference to consult when attempting to handle a routine or problematic request for information, or to familiarize yourself with the major principles associated with the release of medical information.

The potential users of this guide are numerous and diverse: physicians in group or private practice and their employees, hospitals, ambulatory care centers, nursing homes, HMOs, health record professionals, the insurance industry, healthcare and practice management consultants, and students in healthcare administration, allied health, medical assistant, and medical secretarial programs. Regardless of one's professional designation or place of employment, when dealing with release of medical information issues the items of paramount importance are the protection of the patient's right to privacy and the interests of the facility or provider that is releasing the information.

Again, the material presented here is intended to serve only as a quick reference guide for individuals and institutions whose responsibility it is to respond to requests for the release of medical information. In every instance many variables must be considered before releasing otherwise confidential information. Federal and state statutes, facility policy, and legal counsel should always take precedence over this guide.

Users & Uses of Medical Records

Uses of Information in Medical Records

Healthcare Providers — Institutional and Individual (Primary Users)

As a medium of communication among healthcare providers during the current episode of treatment/illness

For facilitating continuity of care

As a reference for future treatment

For training physicians and other personnel, and to assist students in relating theory with medical practice

For prospective and retrospective evaluation of the quality of patient care through review and analysis of patterns of care as documented in the medical record

For promoting effective and efficient use of facilities, equipment, services, personnel, and financial resources through statistical analysis of information abstracted from medical records

For determining and assuring appropriate reimbursement

For documenting voluntary compliance with standards for institutional accreditation

For research aimed at improving treatment, assessing disease detection methods, and assessing the effectiveness of medication and other treatments through study of appropriate cases

For documentation that demonstrates compliance with government regulations

For follow-up care of patients with long-term illnesses and assessing the efficacy of the care given

Payers for Services — Private and Governmental Insurance Plans and Programs and Their Review Organizations (Secondary Users)

For substantiating patient claims for payment of healthcare services

For auditing claims for healthcare services and professional fees

For monitoring the quality, equity, and appropriateness of care and services rendered to those insured

To assess and control the cost of healthcare services to those insured

For developing new plans and programs

Social Users

Public Health Agencies

For surveillance of diseases of epidemiologic significance through statistical analysis of information abstracted from medical records

Medical and Social Researchers — Institutional and Extra-institutional

For investigation of disease patterns and the effects of disease on functions of daily living, including occupational health and safety

Rehabilitation and Social Welfare Programs

For determining need for specific types of rehabilitation programs through analysis of incidence data

For developing individual rehabilitation and training plans for programs for the handicapped and drug and alcohol abusers

Employers

* For administration of employer-provided health insurance plans

* For determining employment suitability

For treatment and analysis of job-related injuries and correction of occupational hazards

For determining disability

Insurance Companies

* For evaluating risks in writing insurance

To determine liability for claims

Government Agencies — Federal, State, and Local

For allocating government resources for schools, healthcare facilities, educational institutions, etc., based on vital statistics submitted from medical records

Education Institutions

* For assessment of suitability for admission to selected educational programs

For maintaining student and employee health programs

Judicial Process

For adjudication of civil and criminal matters using the medical record as evidence through legal process

For involuntary admission of mentally ill

Law Enforcement and Investigation

* In criminal investigations

* For security clearance programs

Credit Investigation Agencies

* For determining credit eligibility

Accrediting, Licensing, and Certifying Agencies

For demonstrating individual fulfillment of requirements of hospital-based education programs

To ascertain competence of practitioners

For documenting compliance with standards for institutional accreditation

For determining compliance with requirements for hospital-based education programs

Media: Press, Radio, TV

For announcing developments in medical research

For reporting health hazards, diseases affecting the public health, and newsworthy events

* This may, in some instances, be an improper use of medical information.

The above information was adapted from "Confidentiality of Patient Health Information: A Position Statement of the American Medical Record Association," *Medical Record News* 49:2 (April 1978): 11–14, and Vicki Carlisle, R.R.A., "Alternative Staffing Services: Correspondence Copiers," *Journal of AHIMA* 63:3 (March 1992): 54–58.

Alphabetical Guide

Press Releases...45

Process (Standard) — for release of information 45

Psychiatric (Mental Health) Records — Release of 45–46

Public Figures — Release concerning...46

Rape Victim — Release concerning 46

Redisclosure of Records...46–47

Refusal to Honor a Request for Information..47

Reportable Diseases, see Diseases — Reportable

Request for the Production of Documents..47–49

Required Reportable Conditions/Incidents..49

Research Studies — Publishing results of...50

Researchers — Release to outside...50

Review of Record...50

Selective Service — Release to...50–51

Service on Which Patient is Hospitalized — Confidentiality of...................................51

Social Service Agencies — Release to...51

Statistical Purposes — Records used for..51

Storage Services, see Contracted Services

Students — Release to...51–52

Subpoenas..52–54

Suicide (Includes Attempted) — Release concerning 55

Telephone Requests...55

Transcription Services, see Contracted Services

Transfer 55–56

    Information to another facility,

    Patient temporarily transferred

Trustees — Release to, see Governing Board of Facility

Venereal Disease 56

Verbal (Oral) Requests 57

Veterans' Administration (VA), see Government Agencies

Voluntary Disclosures..57

Alphabetized Topics

ABORTION — Release where there is evidence of

Whenever documentation in the medical record indicates that an abortion was performed, only the patient may authorize the release of information from that record. This holds true in the case of minors, even in states where parental notification prior to an abortion being performed is required. In some states, however, the treating physician may override the minor's refusal to disclose information if he or she believes it is in the best interest of the minor's physical and mental health.

ABSTRACT

Completing an abstract is one of the best ways to release information from a medical record. An abstract is usually a one-page summary of information extracted from the record that is specific in its response to the request. When providing an abstract in response to a request, file a photocopy of the abstract in the medical record. The practice of completing abstracts is advantageous in that, since only specific information is released, a patient's right to confidentiality is better protected. Also, it is usually much less time consuming than the "photocopying the record" process, especially when there exists an abstract "form" that only needs to be filled in. (See appendix 5)

Notes

ABUSED CHILD REPORTING

Most states have child abuse laws that require any physician or facility having reasonable cause to believe that a child (under a specified age) seen for treatment has suffered injury from physical abuse or neglect inflicted by other than accidental means to report such findings to the designated authority. Although the statutes in most states vary, generally any person having good cause to suspect such abuse is encouraged to report voluntarily. Persons making such reports in good faith are usually protected by statutes from civil or criminal liability.

ACCIDENT VICTIM — Release concerning

When responding to media inquiries concerning an accident victim who has been or who is being treated in the emergency room, several items may be released without the patient's consent (unless the patient has specified otherwise). These items include:

▶ Name

▶ Address

▶ Marital status

▶ Age

▶ Sex

▶ Occupation

▶ General information on the nature of the injuries and the patient's condition

Also, it is always wise to check with the attending physician and law enforcement representatives (if applicable) before releasing information that identifies the patient to the media.

ADDITIONAL INFORMATION FORM

A Request For Additional Information Form may be used when a request for information is received that does not give sufficient information for locating the medical record or contain the proper legal or patient authorization. (See appendix 5.)

ADMINISTRATOR — Release to facility

The facility administrator has free access to all medical records for any facility-related business reason. Except where law or facility policy dictates otherwise, this person makes the final decision as to what medical information may be released and under what circumstances.

AIDS/HIV (Acquired Immune Deficiency Syndrome/Human Immunodeficiency Virus)

AIDS confidential information is that which:

▸ Identifies a person as having been diagnosed with AIDS

▸ Indicates that a person has been or is being treated for AIDS

▸ Indicates that a person is infected with HIV

▸ Reveals that a person has had an HIV test

▸ Reveals that a person has had a positive or negative result to an HIV test

▸ Indicates that a person is considered to be at risk of being infected with AIDS

At present there is much controversy surrounding the AIDS/HIV issue, and there are no hard and fast general rules regarding the release of AIDS/HIV information. Respective state statutes vary *so* greatly that the best advice is to be well versed in your state's tort law regarding this issue and exercise great care in releasing any AIDS-related information. Some states have such restrictive laws and this information is so protected that some providers will not perform an elective HIV test if the patient will not consent to have the information released to an insurer so as to avoid the paperwork nightmare of keeping double billing statements on patients. Conversely, in many states, AIDS/HIV information is afforded no greater protection than the medical record in general. *The best and easiest safeguard is to include a clause specifying the release of AIDS information in a facility's/provider's general authorization form.*

With regard to positive AIDS/HIV test results, they are generally forwarded to the state health department for statistical monitoring, and the patient's identification is not included.

A final note: When in receipt of a request and accompanying authorization that does not specify that the information requested pertains to AIDS/HIV treatment, simply respond by stating that the requestor has not supplied sufficient information for release of the record requested and notify the patient of your action. Do

Notes

the record requested and notify the patient of your action. Do not answer by stating something to the effect that "the authorization that we received from you is not valid for the release of the information you requested." Such a response is a clear indication that the information is of a sensitive and protected nature.

....

AMERICAN ARBITRATION ASSOCIATION

The American Arbitration Association is a public-service, not-for-profit organization dedicated to the voluntary resolution of disputes through the arbitration process. Arbitration is conducted by special rules and procedures, and all parties to the dispute mutually agree to participate in the process and accept the decision of the arbiter(s). Awards/decisions by arbitrators are legally binding and enforceable. Although the Association does not actually decide on cases, it does aid in the administrative process by supplying lists of arbiters from which parties to a dispute mutually select an impartial arbitrator. In its normal course of business, the Association is authorized and may have cause to issue subpoenas duces tecum to aid in the settlement of disputes.

See also: Subpoenas

....

ARMED FORCES — Release to

Requests from the armed forces for medical information must be accompanied by the patient's written authorization. The only information that may be released without the authorization is the patient's name, address, and dates of admission and discharge (the exception to this would be verification of an admission to a facility for treatment of substance and/or alcohol abuse). A provider/facility is not required to release information in the absence of a valid subpoena, court order, or search warrant. If a representative from one of the armed forces wishes to inspect the medical record, the patient's authorization is still required. The individual(s) reviewing the record must present proper identification and must sign and date the patient authorization.

....

ATTORNEYS — Release to

Attorneys have no special privileges when it comes to obtaining confidential medical information — do not be intimidated. Any

Notes

request for information must be accompanied by a valid authorization that includes the patient's signature and specifies the scope (i.e., dates of service) and nature of (especially in cases where psychiatric or substance/alcohol abuse treatment information exists) the information requested and the purpose for which the information is requested. Attorneys have a tendency to request "any and all information." Do not honor such a request.

See also: Redisclosure of Records from Other Facilities/Providers

Subpoenas

Release to Facility Attorney

Although patient authorization is not required, channel requests for medical information from the facility attorney (or the insurer responsible for protecting the facility's interests) through the facility administrator.

AUDITS — Release for financial

There are many instances where a financial audit might be conducted: by agencies concerned with the funding of a facility, review organizations monitoring cost/charge structures and appropriateness of care, claims auditors and tax auditors, grant writers, and so forth. These audits may be specific (e.g., where a specific patient claim has been targeted for review) or general and impersonal (e.g., a review organization monitoring cost of care for specific diagnoses).

Always have external auditors agree, in writing, to conditions that ensure the security and confidentiality of the information, and inform them of the penalty for violating that security — especially where the information is still patient identifiable.

The release of medical information for purposes of audits should be approved by the facility administrator.

AUTHORIZATIONS

Patient

Do not release information from a patient's medical record, except where specified by law or facility policy, without the written authorization of the patient (not his or her spouse), the guardian in case of a minor, the conservator in the case of an incompetent

Notes

person, or executor of the estate, or the next of kin in case of death. As a matter of courtesy, seek the permission of the treating physician when releasing information to a patient.

Contents of a Proper Authorization

Except where otherwise specified by law or (facility) policy, a written authorization by the patient is required prior to the release of medical information. In order for an authorization to be considered valid, it must:

1. Specify the name of the institution releasing the information
2. Specify the name of the individual/agency receiving the information
3. Give the patient's full name, address, and date of birth
4. State the purpose for which the information will be used
5. Specify the extent or nature of the information to be released, including inclusive dates of treatment (requests for "any and all information" should not be honored)
6. Specify the expiration date (or event) of the consent, unless revoked earlier
7. Include a statement to the effect that the consent can be revoked but not retroactive to a release of information made in good faith
8. Be dated (be sure the date of the signature is later than the dates for which the information is to be released)
9. Be signed by the patient (or legal representative)

As added safeguards, it is wise to add two clauses similar to the following to your general authorization form:

▶ A statement that allows the release of AIDS/HIV, mental health, and/or psychiatric information

▶ A statement that releases the treating physician, the facility, and its employees from liability for the release of information made in good faith. (Most states already have laws providing such immunity for a release of information made in good faith and without malice.)

Date and Signature on Authorization

Date

Date authorizations at the time they are signed, and indicate the expiration date on the authorization. In the absence of state laws regarding this issue, the date of expiration should be left to the discretion of the facility. Typically, a consent is not considered valid after one year, the exception being an authorization presented in conjunction with a life or noncancellable, guaranteed renewable health insurance policy (not many of these still in force), in which case the expiration date should not exceed two years from the date of signature. As in all cases, state laws take precedence here, and acceptance of undated consents should be determined by the policy of the facility/provider.

Signature

All authorizations for the release of medical information must be signed by the patient except in a bona fide emergency or if the patient is physically or mentally incompetent, a minor, or deceased. In addition, a signature is not required in cases of permissive disclosure (required or voluntary), such as child abuse reporting or knowledge of juvenile drug use, allowed by respective state laws. Patient signatures on authorizations need not be witnessed by a notary public. If they have not been witnessed, however, they should be compared for authenticity with those found in the medical record (usually on the initial encounter or admissions agreement form).

Authorizations by Those Needing Mental Health Treatment

If a patient has not been adjudicated incompetent by a court, but is only in need of treatment, he or she is still considered competent to sign the necessary authorizations.

Authorizations by Minors

Legally emancipated, married, or those minors who are parents of a child may consent to their own treatment and, as such, are the only ones legally authorized to consent to the release of information from their records. Also, minors who have been treated for venereal disease, contraception, have received an abortion, or who have been treated for alcohol or substance abuse are the only persons able to authorize the release of this type of information. The only exception would be if the treating physician overrides the minor's decision not to release any information, determining it to be in the best interests of the minor's physical and mental health. This provision is specified in many state statutes.

Frequently, the biggest conflict you will encounter when dealing with minors' records is that parents feel they are entitled to the information if they have paid for the services; the fact is, however, they are not.

Authorizations Regarding Deceased

In the case of a deceased patient, the legal representative (estate executor or administrator) signs authorizations for the release of information from the decedent's record. In such cases, it is advisable to obtain either a copy of the Letters of Testamentary (where the deceased left a will) or the Letters of Administration (where the deceased did not leave a will). These documents are issued by the court and indicate that the named individual is the legal representative of the decedent. If there is no legal representative, authorizations may be accepted in the order of priority from individuals in the following list:

1. Spouse

2. Adult son or daughter

3. Either parent

4. Adult brother or sister

5. Any other person authorized or under obligation to dispose of the decedent's body

BIRTH

The details surrounding the birth of a baby (including the fact that a birth has occurred) are confidential. However, many facilities routinely publish a list of recent newborns. Where this practice applies, care should be taken to have the parents sign the necessary release at the time of admission. Obtain the consent of the parents before responding to any inquiries (especially those from the media) concerning a baby's birth.

Birth Certificates

State laws mandate that live births are to be reported to the respective state's center for vital statistics within a specified period of time. Copies of birth certificates should be retained by the hospital, either bound in chronological order or within the individual medical record.

Birth Control — Release where there is evidence of

Whenever documentation in the medical record indicates that an individual has received treatment for birth control, take care to ensure that only the patient authorizes the release of that specific information from the record. This holds true for minors in most states unless the treating physician feels it is in the best interests of the patient's physical or mental health to override the minor's refusal to release such information.

BLUE CROSS/BLUE SHIELD — Release to

The standard Blue Cross/Blue Shield subscription certificate generally requires members to allow access to "all information and records or copies of records for any physician, dentist, podiatrist, nurse, or hospital who has made a diagnosis or treated or rendered service to any beneficiary." The subscriber to the policy agrees on his or her own behalf, and that of any other listed beneficiary, that any of the above mentioned entities are authorized to furnish such information as may be lawful to Blue Cross/Blue Shield upon its request. If the policy is in the patient's name, or if the patient is a minor and the policy is in the guardian's name, no authorization is needed for the release of information. However, if the patient is the spouse of the subscriber, obtain the patient's authorization.

See also: Insurance Companies

BUSINESS OFFICE — Release to facility

Employees in the business office of a facility only have access to those portions of the record containing the applicable information needed for billing, such as the patient's vital information, the insurance subscriber(s) name, address, and employment information, the certificate and group numbers, and a projected length of stay. A primary diagnosis is necessary for pre-certification, and the principal discharge diagnosis would be utilized for the final bill.

In large facilities, requests for more extensive information received from insurance carriers are generally forwarded to the correspondence section of the medical records department. In a provider's office, one person may have the responsibility for billing and releasing information.

Anyone involved with the billing process should see that the necessary information is gathered and that the blanket authorization and assignment of benefits is signed at the time of admission or first patient care encounter. It is usually more difficult to gather needed pieces of information not gathered at the outset.

CHARGES (FEES) — for release of information

A facility or provider is under no obligation to provide free services with regard to the provision/copying of medical information for purposes other than direct patient care. Set a reasonable fee for copying information from the record, for the completion of abstracts, and for record searches. Professional courtesy generally dictates that physicians/facilities are not charged for records requested for purposes of continuity of care. Also, it is never prudent to charge an insurer from whom you are attempting to get reimbursement.

A customary fee is $1 per page, up to a "reasonable" limit (for illustrative purposes, $75). Always let requestors know ahead of time how much the cost will be so they can amend the request if necessary. This may also save you from making unnecessary copies. Set a standard amount for completing abstracts (perhaps $15 to $25), and set an hourly amount (for example, $20) for record searches.

COMMITTEES — Medical staff

Access to Information

Records needed by standing committees of the medical staff for the evaluation of the quality of care are available without the patient's consent.

Confidentiality of Reports

Reports or any other data compiled by in-house staff committees of accredited facilities (including tissue, medical records, medical audit, credentials, utilization review, quality assurance, and risk management, etc.) are confidential and are not usually admissible as evidence in any court action or before any tribunal, board, agency, or person. Medical staff committee reports compiled for the purpose of evaluating the quality of care are definitely hearsay because they are not made in "the regular course of business." They are usually made after the fact in conjunction with the detection of some problem. All the pertinent medical facts needed by attorneys and/or the courts are available in the medical records.

....

CONTRACTED SERVICES

Inclusive in the term "contracted services" are computer services, microfilming companies, storage services, laboratories, data processing firms, transcription, and copying services. All contracted services that process patient-identifiable information for a facility/provider should agree in writing to conditions that:

1. Ensure the security of the information
2. Specify the methods by which the information is to be handled/transported/destroyed
3. Limit and specify the number of types of individuals who: a) have access to the information, and b) are directly involved in the processing of the information, and
4. Specify the penalty for any violation of security or confidentiality

....

CORRESPONDENCE — in the medical record

Historically, correspondence pertaining to a patient has been placed in the medical record to facilitate retrieval of the information. Although correspondence does not usually fall under the category of "medical information," many states have changed their laws to stipulate that all documents found in the medical record relating to the release of information are considered a part of that record. Consult respective state laws when preparing a record in response to a court order or subpoena to see if the correspondence remains with the record or is removed before taking the record to court. Generally speaking, when responding to "informal" requests, i.e., those daily requests made by providers, insurers, etc., do not release correspondence unless your state statute and the request stipulate that you do so.

....

COURT ORDER

A court order is the one request for a medical record that cannot be refused; to do so places one in contempt of court. Prepare

Notes

records in the same manner as if preparing them in response to a subpoena. *Release of substance abuse information requires a special court order.*

See also: Subpoenas

CRIMINALS — Release of records pertaining to

Policy/law with regard to this issue can differ between state and federal institutions. Although most states generally hold that individuals sentenced to penal institutions have lost their civil rights, it is still customary (and advisable) though not always required for prisoners to authorize any release of information. However, prisoners incarcerated in federal prisons still have control over the release of medical information from their records, so authorizations are needed. If an individual is merely being detained in a penal/correctional institution, an authorization is needed before information can be released from his or her medical record.

CUSTODIAN

A custodian is one who has assumed the charge and care of a minor because the parent(s) or legally appointed guardian has died, is in prison, has been adjudicated incompetent, has been committed to an institution, or has deserted the minor and his or her whereabouts are unknown.

DEATH — Release upon occurrence of

Unlike the news of a birth, news of a death is public information. Physicians can release information pertaining to the cause of death. In a medical examiner's case, the general circumstances may be explained, but only the medical examiner is authorized to give the cause of death.

Fetal Death Reporting

File fetal death certificates with the state center for vital statistics within the time period mandated by state law.

Maternity Death Reporting

Report maternity deaths (normal pregnancy, ectopic pregnancy, abortion, and the like) to your respective state health department.

Also, it is customary to report the death of any woman who expires within 90 days of the termination of a pregnancy.

DISCHARGE SUMMARY

Medical information may be and often is released from the medical record in the form of a photocopy of the patient's discharge summary. When releasing information in this manner, as with any release, make note of it in the patient's medical record.

DISEASES — Reportable

In most states, a physician may be responsible for reporting the occurrence of the following diseases:

Amebiasis

Anthrax (in man or animal)

Botulism

Brucellosis (Malta Fever) (in man or animal)

Cat Scratch Fever (in man or animal)

Chancroid

Cholera

Diarrhea of Newborns

Diphtheria

Encephalitis (in man or animal)

Food Poisoning

Glanders (in man or animal)

Gonorrhea

Granuloma Inguinali

Hepatitis, Viral (infectious or serum)

Histoplasmosis

Lead Poisoning

Leprosy

Leptospirosis (Weil's diseases) (in man or animal)

Lymphogranuloma Venereum

Malaria

Meningitis

Meningocemia

Meningococcal Infection

Mumps

Plague

Poliomyelitis

Psittacosis (in man or animal)

Q Fever (in man or animal

Rabies (in man or animal)

Relapsing Fever

Rocky Mountain Spotted Fever

Rubella (congenital)

Salmonellosis (typhoid or paratyphoid)

Shigellosis

Smallpox

Staphylococcus Infection, Newborn

Syphilis

Tetanus

Trichinosis

Tuberculosis (in man or animal)

Tularemia (in man or animal)

Typhus Fever

Whooping Cough

Yellow Fever

Reports of AIDS/HIV positive test results are commonly sent, for statistical monitoring purposes, to state health departments, but they are not patient identifiable.

See also: Required Reportable Conditions/Incidents

AIDS/HIV

Reportable Newborn Conditions

Most states require physicians to report the following newborn diseases/conditions: AIDS/HIV, diarrhea, drug addiction, impetigo, ophthalmia, neonatorum, syphilis, staphylococcus, and PKU.

Notes

DRUG AND ALCOHOL ABUSE RECORDS

Confidentiality

The *Federal Register* of June 9, 1987, effective August 10, 1987, states that records relating to the diagnosis, treatment, rehabilitation, or referral of drug and alcohol abuse patients are considered confidential and can be disclosed only as the regulations stated therein allow; unconditional compliance is required. The federal rules and regulations apply to all programs and activities related to drug or alcohol abuse training, education, treatment, rehabilitation, or research.

Facilities and Programs Affected

The facilities and programs that must comply with federal law when releasing medical information are (1) those conducted in whole or in part (by grant or by contract) by any federal agency, (2) those licensed, registered, or otherwise authorized by a federal agency, (3) those assisted by federal funds, and (4) those assisted by the Internal Revenue Service through tax-exempt status or income tax deductions

Facilities that do not have specialized substance or alcohol abuse treatment programs, but that provide such care incidental to general medical care, are not affected by the regulations. Also, the regulations on confidentiality do not apply to records of those in the armed forces. Military personnel are subject to the Uniform Code of Military Justice (UCMJ). However, any exchange of information must occur exclusively between the various branches of the armed forces or between the armed forces and the Veterans' Administration.

Release to Attorneys

If the patient retains legal counsel, the patient must authorize the release of any information to the attorney. This authorization should also be endorsed by the attorney.

Responding to Subpoena

A subpoena is not sufficient for disclosure of these records. *Drug and alcohol abuse records may only be disclosed pursuant to a court order*, and then only if a hearing indicates that good cause exists for the order. Reasons for disclosure include:

▸ Some noncriminal purposes such as the right of financial recovery by an agency over a "chargeable" entity (i.e., anyone having the ability or obligation to pay a claim)

▸ To investigate or prosecute a patient for an extremely serious crime

▸ To investigate or prosecute a person or program holding the records

▸ To enable the placement of undercover agents or informants for criminal investigation of employees or agents of a program

Contents of Valid Consent

A valid consent from the patient for the release of information pertaining to drug and/or alcohol abuse must contain the following information:

1. A general designation of the program allowed to make the disclosure, thereby eliminating the need to sign multiple consent forms to obtain release of all records from multiple facilities

2. The name of the person/organization authorized to receive the information

3. The patient's name

4. The purpose or need for the disclosure

5. The extent or nature of the information to be released

6. A statement allowing for the revocation of the consent (not retroactive)

7. A specific date or event at which time the consent expires

8. The date it was signed

9. The patient's signature

Criminal Justice System Referrals

Patients being treated for drug and alcohol abuse as a condition of either release from confinement, disposition of criminal proceedings, or a courtimposed sentence can consent to unrestricted disclosure of information by the treatment facility to the court granting probation, the parole board, or probation or parole officer.

Patients being treated as a condition of probation, parole, or release from confinement cannot revoke consent for the unlimited disclosure until there has been a formal termination of the specified situation.

Notes

Release to Third-Party Payers

The disclosure of medical information on drug and alcohol abuse patients can only be made with the individual patient's authorization. Disclosure to third-party payers is limited to that information necessary to fulfill the legal or contractual obligations for payment.

Disclosure Without Consent

Information may be released from a drug and alcohol abuse record without the patient's consent in the following instances:

- ▶ When information is released to medical personnel to meet a bona fide emergency
- ▶ For research activities
- ▶ For governmental and nongovernmental audits and evaluations

Release to Employers

Employers have no access to information contained within an employee's medical record without a valid patient consent.

Acknowledgement of Enrollment in Program

Enrollment/admission to an inpatient facility for drug or alcohol abuse treatment can only be acknowledged to visitors/callers with the patient's written consent. The presence of the patient may be acknowledged if the patient is being treated for a variety of conditions and the response does not indicate that the patient is being treated for drug or alcohol abuse.

Release to Patient's Family

Information concerning the status of the patient may only be disclosed to those parties or individuals related to or having a personal relationship with the patient upon receipt of the patient's written authorization.

Incompetent Patients

If a patient has been adjudicated incompetent, the patient's legal guardian must sign any authorization for the release of medical information.

Minor Patients

The consent of both the minor patient and the parent or guardian is required for the release of information. In states that allow drug and alcohol abuse treatment for minors without parental consent, only the minor's consent is required.

Prohibition on Redisclosure

A statement (amended from the previous regulation to allow for redisclosure with express written consent of the patient) to the following effect must accompany any written disclosure from a drug or alcohol abuse patient's record:

"The enclosed information has been disclosed to you from records whose confidentiality is protected by federal law. Federal regulations prohibit the redisclosure of the information without the written consent of the person to whom it pertains unless further disclosure is expressly permitted by the written consent of the person to whom it pertains. A general authorization for the release of medical information is not sufficient."

Traveling/Incarcerated Patients on Medication

For drug or alcohol abuse patients away from the treatment program and unable to forward an authorization, the treatment program may verify the patient's status within the program and send to the attending medical personnel the information needed for treatment. This can be done only after the attending medical personnel have assured those acting on the treatment program's behalf that the patient has requested medication and has consented to the release of information. When making disclosures of this kind, document the patient's name, patient's number, date and time of disclosure, the information disclosed, to whom it was disclosed, and the name of the discloser.

A final note: When in receipt of a request and accompanying authorization that does not specify that the information requested pertains to treatment of drug and alcohol abuse, simply respond by stating that the requestor has not supplied sufficient information for release of the record requested and notify the patient of your action. Do not answer by stating something to the effect that "the authorization that we received from you is not valid for the release of the information you requested." Such a response is a clear indication that the information is of a sensitive and protected nature.

EMANCIPATED MINORS

In the majority of states a minor who is married, the parent of a child, lives apart from parents, and is self-supporting is considered "emancipated." An emancipated minor has the same capacity as an adult to consent to treatment and, as such, is the only person able to authorize the release of information from his or her medical record.

ETHICS: THE ISSUE OF CONFIDENTIALITY

The Hippocratic Oath is generally considered the source of principles and ethics as they relate to the confidentiality of medical information: "Whatsoever I shall see or hear concerning the life of men, in my attendance on the sick or even apart therefrom which ought not be noised abroad, I will keep silence thereon, counting such things as holy secrets." Patients, knowing that the information revealed to a physician remains confidential, are thereby encouraged to make candid disclosures, which promotes the ability of the physician to diagnose and treat. Therefore, ethical obligations dictate that a physician hold confidential any information obtained from patients unless required by law to reveal the information, or if the release of information is necessary to protect the welfare of an individual or the community. Although not bound by an oath, all ancillary healthcare providers are generally considered to be accountable for the adherence to this code of ethics.

EXTENDED CARE FACILITY — Release to

When a patient is transferred to an extended care facility, no authorization is needed for the release of information. The transferring facility's report should include current medical findings, diagnosis, rehabilitation potential, discharge summary, nursing and dietary information, ambulation status, and relevant administrative and social information.

FAX (FACSIMILE) MACHINE — Release by

Transmit medical information by fax only when the information is needed for a patient care encounter and the original record or mail-delivered photocopies would not reach the recipient in a timely manner. Do not respond to routine requests for medical information from insurance companies, attorneys, or other nonhealthcare entities by fax; use regular mail or courier service.

When transmitting information by fax, obtain a properly executed patient authorization prior to the release of the information. It is acceptable to honor an authorization transmitted by fax. Observe the following procedures when transmitting or receiving medical information by fax.

Sending ("Faxing") Information

1. Attach a cover letter including the following information:
   - Date and time of fax transmission
   - Sending facility's name and address
   - Sending facility's telephone and facsimile number
   - Sender's name
   - Receiving facility's name, telephone, and facsimile number
   - Authorized receiver's name
   - Number of copies sent (including cover letter)
   - Statement regarding redisclosure
   - Statement regarding destruction (or return fax received in error)
   - Instructions for authorized receiver to verify receipt of information
2. Verify by telephone the availability of the authorized receiver to receive the information prior to beginning the transmission
3. Document the fact of the transmission by fax in your correspondence log
4. File the original cover letter in the correspondence section of the medical record
5. Request that the authorized receiver sign and return the attached receipt form upon receipt of the information

Ideally, a statement to the following effect should appear at the bottom of your fax cover sheet:

Notice

Unauthorized interception of this telephonic communication could be a violation of federal and state law(s).

The documents attached to this transmittal contain confidential information. They belong to the sender and are legally privileged.

The information contained herein is intended for use only by the authorized receiver named above. It cannot be redisclosed for use by any other party. If you are not the authorized receiver you are hereby notified that any disclosure, copying, distribution, or taking any action in reliance on the information contained herein is prohibited. If you have received these documents in error, notify the sender immediately by telephone to arrange for the return of or instructions for destruction of the original documents to said sender.

Receiving Information

1. Authorize one person to be responsible for monitoring the fax machine

2. Remove faxed documents from the tray immediately upon completion of transmission

3. Count the number of pages received

4. Read the cover letter and follow any instructions contained therein

5. Notify the authorized receiver that a fax has been received

6. Seal the documents in an envelope and hold for pick-up (if the person monitoring the fax is not the authorized receiver)

In case of a misdirected fax, fax a notice explaining the situation and ask that the information received be returned by mail or destroyed. Automatic dialing features in some machines can help prevent the problem of misdirected faxes. Another safeguard is to photocopy any documents faxed on thermal paper prior to their being filed in the medical record. Thermal paper has a tendency to deteriorate over time.

For further information regarding this current issue, consult: Laura Feste, "Practice Bulletin: Guidelines for Faxing Patient Health Information." *Journal of the American Medical Record Association* 62:6 (June 1991): 29–32.

GOVERNING BOARD OF FACILITY — Release to

Channel requests by board members for use of medical records or the release of information through the facility administrator.

GOVERNMENT AGENCIES — Release to

Requests from government agencies and representatives (state and national) for medical information must be accompanied by the patient's written authorization. The only information that may be released without the authorization is the patient's name and address and dates of admission and discharge (the exception would be admission to a facility for treatment of drug and/or alcohol abuse). Facilities are not required to release information in the absence of a subpoena. The representative(s) of a government agency wishing to review the record must present proper identification and must sign and date the patient's authorization. Such agencies include:

▸ Federal Bureau of Investigation (FBI)

▸ Internal Revenue Service (IRS)

▸ Armed Forces

▸ Veterans' Administration (VA)

▸ Selective Service/Draft Boards/Induction Centers

▸ National Labor Relations Board

▸ Social Security Administration (SSA)

▸ Railroad Commission

These agencies have the power to subpoena; when in receipt of a subpoena, consider the nature of the information cited before complying with the demand.

IMPERSONAL DOCUMENT — Use of record as

A medical record may be used as an impersonal document by medical staff members for research and study, presentations, and conferences; by residents and interns for research, training, and study; by nurses and other paramedical personnel for case studies and training; financial auditors; and by outside researchers. Patient authorization is not required for such uses of the medical record. Requests for information from external auditors and researchers, however, should be channeled through the facility administrator. Any outside party that is given access to patient identifiable information must agree in writing to conditions that ensure the security of the information and specify the penalty for violating that confidentiality.

INCOMPETENT DRIVERS' ACT

Many states have the equivalent of an incompetent drivers' act, which defines the disabilities and circumstances for which a person's license to drive may be limited or revoked. A physician may voluntarily report the finding of such a disability to the appropriate agency. The information usually included in such a report is the patient's name, date of birth, address, and the disability which would prevent a driver from safely operating a motor vehicle.

....

INSURANCE COMPANIES

Acting as Third-Party Payers

Releasing medical information to private insurance companies requires the patient's written authorization. Release only that information specifically requested and only for the period of hospitalization specified in the patient's authorization. In the absence of a request for specific information, the following information may be released: dates of admission and discharge, final diagnosis, the type and date of surgery (if any was performed), and the names of the attending physician and surgeon(s). It is best to discourage requests for "any and all information."

Current theory and practice indicates that facilities and providers need not be overly concerned about the consequences of releasing information to insurance companies specifically designated by patients as their third-party payers; patients generally sign a blanket authorization upon admission or first patient encounter allowing the release of information and assignment of benefits. When following a less stringent process to expedite claims processing and payment by the carriers, remember to use any special consent forms required by law, state or federal, or to provide for records of a protected nature (e.g., alcohol and substance abuse records, AIDS/HIV records, mental health/psychiatric records, etc.) in your general authorization.

Representing Physicians

Patient authorization need not necessarily accompany a request from an agent of the physician's malpractice carrier. Consult your respective state statute and/or attorney when in receipt of such a request. It is generally accepted that a patient has waived the right to confidentiality by becoming a party to a malpractice suit.

Representing Facilities

In that they are protecting the interests of the facility (or provider), requests from insurers in this instance do not require the patient's authorization to release the requested information.

INTERHOSPITAL AGREEMENTS

Metropolitan hospitals often establish interhospital agreements that allow for the rapid exchange of information needed for patient care. Although most state laws provide for the release of information without patient consent if it is necessary for direct patient care, participating hospitals are advised to obtain the patient's consent to such an arrangement prior to or at the time of admission to avoid the possibility of any legal consequences.

See also: Transfer of Information to Another Facility

Transferred, Patient Temporarily

INTOXICATED PERSON — Release regarding

Refer requests for information concerning patients treated for intoxication to the police (especially in the case of requests from the media). Otherwise, withhold the information in the absence of the patient's written authorization.

JUVENILE DRUG USE

Many state statutes encourage that voluntary disclosure of suspected habitual use of marijuana or other controlled substances by a juvenile be made by any interested party having knowledge of such drug use to a designated authority or agency. Those persons making such reports in good faith are usually protected by statute from civil or criminal liability.

LAWSUIT — Patient bringing

Whenever a patient, as plaintiff, initiates a lawsuit based on a claim of malpractice, full compliance with the demands of those requiring to see and copy the pertinent records (i.e., physician's and/or facility's attorneys and insurers) is understood to be a condition of that action.

See also: Malpractice

LOG — Release of information

A log of information released, usually referred to as a correspondence log, serves as a continuous record of information that has been and is being released and to whom. It also serves as a tool for measuring the correspondence workload within a medical record department. Information contained in the log should include:

► Patient name and number

► Date request received

► To whom it was assigned

► Name of requestor

► Type of information requested

► Type of information mailed

► Reason request denied — if applicable

► Date that any correspondence pertaining to request was sent

► Processing charges and paid/unpaid status

MALPRACTICE — Review of record in event of

In the event of a malpractice or professional negligence suit against a physician and/or a facility, review the medical record in question for completeness, timeliness of entries, relevance, accuracy, legibility, and comprehensibility. Ideally, this review should be a cooperative effort between the attending physician, the medical record administrator, the facility administrator, and the facility attorney. Pending any legal action, it is a good idea to remove the record from the general file — take it out of circulation, so to speak — to ensure its integrity.

MEDICAID (MEDICAL ASSISTANCE) — Release to

It is generally accepted that requests from Medicaid may be honored without the specific written authorization of the patient, as such authorization is a condition of coverage. The rules governing Medicaid call for the routine disclosure of medical information by a provider or facility specifically for the purpose of processing claims under the program.

See also: Medicare

MEDICAL EXAMINER — Release to

Once a body has been released to the medical examiner, confidential information pertaining to the decedent may also be released to authorized persons in that office. Verify the requestor's position with said office. Request a subpoena if you have any doubt about the validity of a request.

MEDICAL INFORMATION BUREAU

The Medical Information Bureau is a nonprofit membership organization of life insurance companies that allows for information exchange, specifically claims and medical history information, between member companies. It operates similarly to a credit bureau. When an individual applies to a Bureau member for life or health coverage or submits a claim for benefits to a member company, the Bureau, upon request, supplies information in its file pertaining to that individual. An individual may request and receive access to any of his or her information on file with the Bureau. Corrections may be made to one's file in accordance with procedures set forth in the Federal Fair Credit Reporting Act. The Bureau's address is:

P. O. Box 105

Essex Station

Boston, MA 02112

(617) 426-3660

MEDICARE — Release to

Medicare is much like Medicaid in that the routine disclosure of medical information pertinent to claims processing is a condition of coverage. A patient usually signs a pre-admission or patient information form upon his or her first patient care encounter authorizing the release of information to the Medicare intermediary as well as the assignment of benefits. The statement generally reads, "I authorize any holder of medical or other information about me to release to the Social Security Administration or its intermediaries any information needed for this or a related Medicare claim. I request that payment of authorized benefits be made on my behalf."

MICROFILMED RECORDS — Legal acceptance of

In 1951 the United States Senate recognized the reliability of the microfilm process in Senate Report no. 537, which recommended the passage of the Uniform Photographic Copies of Business and Public Records as Evidence Act (UPA). With regard to medical records, the UPA authorizes the destruction of an original record after copying if the destruction is in the regular course of business and is not in violation of a statutory duty to preserve the original. This act is recognized in most states.

NONCONFIDENTIAL INFORMATION

The following information is generally considered nonconfidential and may be released without the patient's specific consent unless otherwise specified by the patient or the facility. As always, care should be taken to verify the legitimacy of an inquiry. The information that may be released includes:

- ▸ Name
- ▸ Address at time of admission (address at time of discharge may be confidential)
- ▸ Age and sex
- ▸ Occupation/employer
- ▸ Dates of admission and discharge
- ▸ Verification of hospitalization
- ▸ General condition upon discharge (alive or dead)

The exceptions to the above are for drug or alcohol abuse patients and cases wherein the patient or his or her legal representative has stipulated that the information not be released.

NURSING HOME RESIDENT ABUSE — Reporting of

Most states have laws that require anyone having knowledge of the abuse or exploitation of a resident of a nursing home or long-term care facility to report the situation immediately to the appropriate agency, usually the Department of Human Resources or its equivalent. Situations requiring reporting include assault or battery, failure to provide treatment or care, sexual harassment, seemingly improper use of a patient or of the patient's property for profit, gross negligence, and so forth. States having such a law usually provide for the protection of the person making a report in good faith. These laws usually extend to include protection from retaliatory or discriminatory acts directed at the person making the disclosure and/or the object of the report by the facility.

OTHER HEALTHCARE FACILITIES — Release to

Medical information may be released to other healthcare facilities only upon receipt of the patient's written authorization. The exception is a bona fide emergency situation, in which the "call back procedure" is followed (see Telephone Requests). Also, no authorization is necessary if the information being released is to an extended care facility, nursing home, or acute care facility to which the patient is being transferred. See Extended Care Facility.

OWNERSHIP OF RECORD

The physical medical record is the property of the facility or provider. It is kept for the benefit of the patient, the medical staff, and the facility. The information contained within the record belongs to the patient and cannot be released, unless otherwise specified, without the written consent of the patient, the issuance of a subpoena or court order, or the presence of a state statute or federal law.

PATIENT — Release to

State statutes vary widely with regard to patients having access to their medical records. Most states (in keeping with the general trend toward consumer rights) have mandated that the patient should have free access to the medical record; others have left it to the discretion of the respective facilities and providers. The Privacy Act, which prevails in federal institutions, not only gives the patient access to the record, but allows the patient to correct and/or amend it. Whatever the law may be for a given state, it is good practice to refer all patient requests to see and copy their records to the attending physician or the chief medical officer of the facility.

If the physician determines that access to the record would be detrimental to the mental or physical well-being of the patient, make notation of that determination in the chart. Some states require that if patient access is denied, the information must be released to another patient-designated provider. Consider the following when responding to a patient request:

- ▶ Nature of information in the record
- ▶ Purpose for which access is sought
- ▶ Rights and best interests of patient, physician, and facility
- ▶ Legal requirements

PERSONNEL OF HEALTHCARE FACILITY — Release to

Inclusive in the term "personnel" are residents, interns, and nurses. Personnel have no special privileges per se, but they may inspect patient records when necessary for carrying out their routine work, inspect their own records upon presenting a written request, and inspect the medical records of relatives only upon receipt of the patient's written authorization.

PHOTOCOPIES OF RECORDS

Photocopies are the common and sometimes most practical way to respond to a request. A prepaid fee is usually required of the requestor. Remind the receiving party in writing that the information is confidential and is to be used only for the purpose for which it was requested and not redisclosed (see Redisclosure) to another facility or provider in the absence of the patient's specific written authorization, a subpoena, or a court order. There are "correspondence copying" companies that contract with facilities and providers to aid in processing large volumes and/or backlogs of requests.

PHYSICIANS — Releasing Information to

Company

It is permissible to transfer medical information to a company-employed physician caring for a patient following discharge from a hospital or other treatment facility (exceptions include facilities for psychiatric treatment or treatment for substance or alcohol abuse). Such information is not accessible to the company's personnel department or management.

Notes

Staff

A staff physician only has access to the records of those patients he or she is currently treating. If a patient is readmitted to the facility under the care of another physician, all records are immediately available to the present attending physician.

Nonstaff

A patient must authorize the release of medical information to a physician who is not on the medical staff of the facility that houses the record. Although there are some states whose permissive disclosure laws allow for the release of information to a physician or provider who requests the information stating that the patient is currently under his or her care, an oral or written request signed by the provider and accompanied by the patient's written authorization is the most widely practiced and accepted procedure.

Referring

At the request of a staff physician, an abstract of medical information may be sent without the patient's consent to a referring physician who is not a member of the medical staff.

Releasing Name

Although not classified as confidential information, always obtain the consent of the physician before including his or her name in any media releases. It is also wise to use caution when disclosing the name of a physician who is specifically affiliated with the treatment of alcohol and/or substance abuse or psychiatric care.

PHYSICIANS — Improper acts

Each state has the equivalent of a Medical Practice Act that allows a state board of medical examiners to refuse a license to practice medicine or to discipline a physician who already holds a license. Generally included in these acts is the provision allowing anyone to make a good faith report of questionable practices (acts or omissions) by a physician. The provisions of these acts further protect the reporting party from civil or criminal liability.

PKU SCREENING — Reports on newborns discharged without

Periodic reports on newborns discharged alive without having had a PKU (phenylketonuria) screening are generally made to state health departments.

PRESS RELEASES

One or more persons within a facility should be designated to handle all information requests from the media. These people must be thoroughly briefed on state laws and facility policy with regard to media inquiries and the release of medical information. Make the names of those persons designated known to telephone operators, admissions, the information desk, the emergency room, and, if the function is not already lodged in that location, the medical record department. In short, *any* location likely to receive calls from the media.

PROCESS (STANDARD) — for release of information

Although no process is foolproof, it is extremely good practice to have a clear procedure to follow when releasing information to third parties. A process that reminds you to check for a current patient authorization, that the request itself is valid, that federal and state confidentiality laws and guidelines are followed, and so forth will help ensure that the release of information is properly handled. For that purpose, we have included a checklist in appendix 5 for releasing information.

PSYCHIATRIC (MENTAL HEALTH) RECORDS — Release of

Always use great care and caution when releasing information of this sensitive nature and know your respective state's law and facility's policy regarding these types of records. In some states, the mention of a psychiatric diagnosis incidental to other medical care is not afforded any greater protection than that given to medical information in general; a record generated by a psychiatric or mental health provider, however, is afforded extra protection — the "authorship" of the information is the deciding factor. In other states, the mere mention of a psychiatric diagnosis is granted special protection. Suffice it to say, this information is and should be carefully guarded. *The best safeguard is to include a clause in your general authorization statement covering the release of psychiatric/mental health information.*A final note: When in receipt of a request and accompanying authorization that does not specify that the information requested pertains to treatment of psychiatric cases, simply respond by stating that the requestor has not supplied sufficient information.

PUBLIC FIGURES — Release concerning

A hospital may confirm that a public figure is hospitalized unless such confirmation has been forbidden by the patient or the patient's physician. Where widespread interest exists, the attending physician(s) may arrange for the release of periodic bulletins on the patient's status.

RAPE VICTIM — Release concerning

In many states, medical information pertaining to a rape may only be released to law enforcement representatives if the victim has consented to such release by deciding to proceed with the legal process. It is a good idea to refer any inquiries concerning a rape victim to the police.

REDISCLOSURE OF RECORDS

Copies of medical information/records from other facilities or providers that have been incorporated into the patient's medical record do not become the property of the receiving party. Do not photocopy and send them to a third party without the written consent of the patient. Facilities or providers responding to a request for information should attach a Redisclosure Statement to the information being released. The statement should read: "The enclosed information has been disclosed to you from records whose confidentiality is protected. This information is not to be disclosed to a third party without the express written consent of the person to whom it pertains." On the rare occasion an entire patient record must be released, include a cover letter that states, "the enclosed records are all the records from our facility." This lets the requestor (an attorney or legal body, most frequently) know that all the information in the file has not been sent. The requestor can then, if desired, subpoena any information from other facilities or providers contained in the file.

Notes

REFUSAL TO HONOR A REQUEST FOR INFORMATION

A facility or provider, upon the advice of legal counsel, can refuse to honor the written authorization of a patient and compel a court to rule on the request for medical information if it is felt that honoring the request would not be in the best interests of the patient, physician, or facility. The following conditions are generally applicable to a refusal:

1. Reasonable doubt exists as to the identity of the person presenting the authorization

2. There is evidence that the party requesting the information is not identical to the party named in the authorization

3. Evidence indicates that the patient is not of legal age

4. There is a question concerning the patient's mental capacity to know that he or she signed the authorization

5. No verification is present that the person signing for a minor or incompetent person is legally qualified to do so

6. The authenticity of the signature is suspect

7. Disclosure would be detrimental to the physical or mental well-being of the patient

8. Disclosure may cause the patient to harm himself or herself or someone else

REQUEST FOR THE PRODUCTION OF DOCUMENTS

A Request for the Production of Documents is an increasingly popular method used by attorneys pursuing the discovery process in a lawsuit to obtain pertinent medical information. (In some states a "Request for the Production of Documents" is synonymous with "Subpoena" and handled accordingly – see also subpoena). These requests usually specifically identify the documents to be inspected and the manner (i.e., date, time, place) in which they will be inspected.

The following characteristics make complying with this type of request cumbersome and confusing:

▸ A Request for the Production of Documents may be served on those who have no involvement in a suit as well as those who are a party to the litigation

▸ All parties to the litigation must be afforded the same opportunity to inspect the documents as the requesting party

▶ Compliance with this type of request is costly and inconvenient if the request stipulates that the documents be presented and copied at the office of the attorney making the request

▶ In many states, a Request for Production of Documents means to produce the original documents (unlike statutes pertaining to subpoenas), which means the original medical record might be removed from the facility's premises

▶ It can be difficult and expensive to copy and route the requested information to all parties to the litigation

▶ The patient may not be aware of the request and thus have no opportunity to file a formal objection if he or she is not a party to the litigation

The easiest way to resolve this potentially undesirable situation is to ask (persuade) the requesting attorney to make the request by subpoena. If this is not possible, the following is a suggested procedure for complying with a Request for the Production of Documents:

1. Ascertain whether the patient is a party to the action.

   ▶ If the patient appears to be a party to the suit, wait to see if the patient, through his or her attorney, objects to the production of documents; if not, comply with the request.

   ▶ If it appears the patient is not a party to the suit, notify him or her of the request, thereby providing the opportunity to object.

   (Send a form letter to the patient immediately upon receipt of the request, thereby eliminating the need for determining if the patient is indeed a party to the suit.)

2. Review the stipulations cited in the request. Often, if production of the record is required elsewhere other than the facility's premises, delivery of a certified copy is deemed sufficient compliance.

   ▶ If such is not the case, involve the facility attorney in an effort to resolve the matter in a friendly and mutually satisfactory manner (i.e., a request by subpoena).

   ▶ Deliver a certified copy of the record to the requestor's office, if acceptable.

   ▶ If the facility is designated as the site for the inspection and no objections surface, make the record(s) available at the date and time specified.

▸ Include a fee for copying when delivering a copy of the record.

▸ Consult the facility attorney regarding any irregularities noted in a request.

* H. Boyce Connell, Jr., *The Georgia Law of Medical Records*, rev. ed. (Atlanta: Georgia Medical Record Association, 1987): 49–51.

REQUIRED REPORTABLE CONDITIONS/INCIDENTS

In complying with various state statutes, the conditions and/or incidents that a knowledgeable and responsible person may be required to report include:

Child abuse (disclosure may be voluntary)

Communicable diseases in dead bodies

Fetal deaths

Gunshot wounds

Injuries caused by knives, ice picks, and other sharp instruments

Juvenile drug abuse (disclosure usually voluntary)

Machinery accidents (e.g., lawn mower)

Nonaccidental injuries

Nursing home resident abuse (disclosure may be voluntary)

Spinal cord disabled/head injured

Unusual/suspicious deaths

Venereal/communicable diseases (disclosure may be voluntary)

See also: Diseases, Reportable

RESEARCH STUDIES — Publishing results of

Do not release the results of research studies without the permission of the attending physician(s).

RESEARCHERS — Release to outside

Information from patient medical records may be used for research purposes without the patient's authorization. The facility administrator and medical staff are responsible for establishing policies for the release of information to outside researchers. Facility policy should specify that requests must (1) be in writing, (2) include the purpose of the project, (3) contain a statement accepting responsibility for the confidentiality of the information and the patients' identities, and (4) be approved by the facility administrator. Do the abstracting at the convenience of the medical record department and charge a fee for it.

REVIEW OF RECORD

Review (inspection) of the medical record is one way to obtain medical information. For example, a medical record is often inspected as a condition of a Request for the Production of Documents. Remember that in the absence of a law or policy dictating otherwise, the patient's written authorization must be obtained prior to any review of the record. The patient's medical record must be reviewed in the presence of either medical record personnel or the attending physician for the case. The reviewer must sign and date the patient's authorization at the time of the review.

See also: Malpractice

Armed Forces

Government Agencies

Selective Service

SELECTIVE SERVICE — Release to

The patient's name, address, and the dates of admission and discharge may be released to the Selective Service (draft board) without the patient's consent (the exception to this would be verification of admission to a facility for treatment of substance or alcohol abuse). The patient's written authorization or a subpoena is needed for the release of other confidential medical information. Selective Service representatives wishing to review a record must present proper identification and sign and date the patient's authorization.

SERVICE ON WHICH PATIENT IS HOSPITALIZED — Confidentiality of

The hospital medical care service on which a patient is hospitalized is confidential information.

SOCIAL SERVICE AGENCIES — Release to

A patient must authorize the release of medical information to any social service agency, caseworkers, and any personnel from agencies such as half-way houses, welfare offices, charities, and so forth.

STATISTICAL PURPOSES—Records used for

Medical records are used as impersonal documents by various entities in compiling healthcare statistics used in planning optimal healthcare system(s).

Statistical analysis is the manner by which epidemiologically significant diseases are tracked, the need for specific types of healthcare programs is determined, the amount of government allocations to healthcare and educational facilities is assessed, and so forth.

As always, when the information is requested for such impersonal use by outside statisticians and researchers, the requestor must agree in writing to conditions that ensure the security and confidentiality of the information and specify the penalty for violating that security. Also, notify the facility administrator of such requests.

STUDENTS — Release to

Students participating in medical or allied health programs affiliated with a facility may have access to the medical records of any patients assigned to them. They may also have access to other records needed for educational and research purposes if the patients have given their actual or implied (by their presence at a teaching facility) consent. A request by a student to review a patient's record after the patient has been discharged may require the authorization of the student's supervisor.

SUBPOENAS

A subpoena is a document issued by a court or other authorized agency or individual requiring the person served to comply with its terms under penalty of law. Many entities have the power to subpoena, including state, superior, probate, and federal courts; attorneys; the American Arbitration Association; workers compensation boards; state boards of medical examiners; coroners' and medical examiners' offices; and the like. When served with a subpoena, always verify the legal authority of the issuing body or party, and whether the scope and terms of the subpoena are sufficient to warrant release of the medical record in question.

Subpoena Duces Tecum

This is the most frequently encountered type of subpoena and is more properly known as a "subpoena for the production of documentary evidence." Such a document requests the production of documents (the medical record) and possibly the attendance of a witness to testify to the manner in which the record(s) was created. The physical presence of the medical record (or a certified copy, if acceptable) will be required in court.

Serving

Respective state statutes determine the manner by which a subpoena may be served. Generally, it is served in person or by certified or registered mail. The subpoena must specify as concisely as possible the records or documents required. The description of the documents does not have to be detailed, just sufficient to identify them with reasonable certainty.

Processing (Preparation of) Documents

The following checklist provides a good review of items to consider when complying with and preparing documents in response to a subpoena:

- ❐ A subpoena duces tecum should be served so as to allow a reasonable amount of time to locate and assemble the required documents.

- ❐ When served with a subpoena, determine whether or not it is a duplicate of one that has already been served. While the server is still present, check for the name and telephone number of the party responsible for the subpoena and the docket number of the case.

❐ Check immediately to see if the patient whose record has been requested has been treated at the facility or by the provider.

❐ Phone the requesting party to determine exactly when you and/or the record are required to appear. (This saves unnecessary time waiting to be called or unnecessary trips if the case is settled or dismissed.)

❐ If the medical record is on microfilm, notify whomever is responsible for the subpoena; they may decide against using the record. If they still wish the record to appear, advise them that they must provide the reader or have diazo copies made at their expense.

❐ Record the receipt of the subpoena in the correspondence log.

❐ Collect the material requested. Consult respective state statutes to see if psychiatric records (notes and consults), correspondence, social service notes, and copies of abstracts and insurance reports should remain with the record or be removed before it is taken to court.

❐ Check the record for completeness and integrity in all respects — all reports and signatures must be present. Bring any discrepancies to the attention of the facility administrator and facility attorney.

❐ Count the pages to be submitted and record the number on a folder. Make duplicate lists of the items in the record. The original list may be signed as a receipt if the medical record must be left in court. Leave the duplicate list in the medical record folder at the facility/office. If the original record is not required, photocopy all those documents to be submitted.

❐ As a matter of courtesy, notify the attending physician of the subpoena duces tecum. Immediate notification is appropriate if the physician is named as a party to litigation.

Delivery of Documents

In the absence of a phrase to the effect that "for good cause shown, the court orders the appearance of the custodian of the records," it is generally understood that the delivery of the original record or a certified copy (if acceptable) to the clerk of the court issuing the subpoena or some other person designated by the subpoena (if legally allowed) constitutes full compliance. In fact, many states now deem certified copies of the medical record an adequate response to a subpoena duces tecum unless otherwise specified. When submitting a certified copy in response

Notes

to a subpoena, attach a certificate of authenticity indicating that the enclosed records are true and accurate copies of the requested medical record(s) signed before a notary public or another individual authorized to administer oaths. Actual delivery can be by any means — in person or by certified or registered mail — which will provide a receipt for delivery.

Review of Record in Court

Neither of the attorneys (representing either the plaintiff or the defendant) should be allowed to review the record except by mutual consent of both attorneys.

As Witness in Court

When required, a witness, usually the custodian of the records, testifies that the medical record was created in the regular course of business and that any person making entries did so as part of his or her usual activity.

Leaving the Record in Court

Allow the original medical record to remain in court only after it has been admitted as evidence and the judge has stipulated that it must remain. In this event, see if it is possible to leave either a certified copy of the original record or a diazo copy if it is a microfilmed record. If copies are not acceptable, obtain a receipt for the original from the clerk of court, the party who initiated the subpoena, or the judge. Follow-up periodically to ensure that the record is returned to the facility/office as soon as possible. *Do not* leave a medical record when answering a deposition subpoena for discovery purposes.

SUICIDES (INCLUDES ATTEMPTED) — Release concerning

Refer inquiries from the media concerning suicides or attempted suicides to the police.

TELEPHONE REQUESTS

Discourage telephone requests for medical information. They should only be honored in bona fide emergency situations. An emergency request is usually placed by a physician or facility who needs the information in order to treat the patient. Handle the request via a "call-back" verification procedure. Simply request the caller's name and number, saying that you will call back with the necessary information. Then call back to verify the identity of the caller and provide or fax the information.

Note: *The above verification procedure should be followed during the routine telephone interchange that so often takes place between facilities/provider offices/labs seeking test results or consult findings.*

Documenting

Document the following (either in a log reserved for that purpose or in the patient's medical record) for all telephone requests:

- ▸ Date of the request
- ▸ Name of the requestor
- ▸ The information requested
- ▸ Patient's name (and patient number)
- ▸ Name of the treating physician
- ▸ The information released
- ▸ To whom the call was referred (if applicable)

TRANSFER

Information to Another Facility

Frequently, patients are discharged from one facility and transferred to another (acute care or skilled nursing facility, home health agency, hospice, nursing home, neighborhood clinic, etc.). No authorization is needed to release information to these facilities when a transfer is taking place. The transferring facility's report should include current medical findings, diagnosis, prognosis, rehabilitation potential, discharge summary, nursing and dietary information, ambulation status, and any relevant administrative and social information.

Patient Temporarily Transferred

When a patient is temporarily transferred to another facility for treatment (e.g., radiation therapy, physical therapy, CT scans, surgery, etc.), the medical record or pertinent portions thereof usually accompany the patient if both institutions agree that all treatment rendered will be reported and retained in the referring facility's medical record. Otherwise, enter into an agreement to the effect that there will be an exchange of pertinent information in each institution's record.

See also: Other Healthcare Facilities

Extended Care Facility

VENEREAL DISEASE

Only the person treated for venereal disease may authorize the release of medical information from that record. This includes minors who have been treated for venereal disease — even though their parents may be paying the bill. The only exception here is if the treating physician overrides the minor's decision not to release the information, determining it to be in the best interest of the minor's physical and mental health.

Further, the mandatory reporting laws of most states universally require the occurrence of diseases such as gonorrhea and syphilis be reported to state health departments. These reports are patient identifiable to allow for follow-up. Many states also require the reporting of positive HIV tests for statistical purposes. Generally, the information in these cases is not patient identifiable.

Most state statutes also have a provision allowing for and encouraging anyone having knowledge of a case of venereal disease to report it to the state health department. Those making such voluntary disclosures in good faith and without fraud or malice are also protected by statute.

See also: Authorization by Minors

Diseases, Reportable

Required Reportable Conditions/Incidents

Voluntary Disclosures

VERBAL (ORAL) REQUESTS

Any person (other than the patient or the patient's legal representative) making a verbal request for medical information, either in person or over the phone, is no different from any other requestor. Do not be intimidated. In the absence of a law or policy dictating otherwise, the patient's written authorization is always required. (This includes the law enforcement officer in full regalia who presents a search warrant or subpoena and demands a patient's drug abuse records — only a special court order releases those records.)

See also: Telephone Request

....

VOLUNTARY DISCLOSURES

Most state statutes have provisions that allow and encourage those persons having knowledge regarding the occurrence of one of the following situations to report this information to a designated agency:

▶ Child abuse

▶ Incompetent drivers (only physicians make these reports)

▶ Juvenile drug use

▶ Nursing home resident abuse

▶ Physician's improper acts

▶ Venereal disease

State statutes allowing voluntary disclosure also protect those making the reports in good faith and without fraud or malice from civil or criminal liability.

....

WORKERS COMPENSATION — Release to

Workers Compensation is administered within each state. Any individual eligible who applies for workers compensation automatically authorizes the release of information specifically related to the treatment of the injury to a workers compensation board or commission. Although no specific authorization is required for the release of information, always verify that the request is part of a workers compensation action by (1) determining if the injury was sustained during working hours by checking the medical record, (2) contacting the facility business office to see if it has a record of the claim, and (3) obtaining a board claim number if it was not already included on the request. The workers compensation boards and/or the workers compensation administrative law judges have the power to subpoena.

Bibliography

Anastasio, Denise. "Current Practices For Release of Medical Information." *Journal of the American Medical Record Association* 61:6 (June 1990): 52–61.

Anthony, Michael. "Issues Relating To Patients' Access to Their Medical Records." *Medical Record News* 48:6 (December 1977): 85–91.

Carlisle, Vicki. "Alternative Staffing Services: Correspondence Copiers." *Journal of AHIMA* 63:3 (March 1992): 54–58.

"Confidentiality of Patient Health Information: A Position Statement of the American Medical Record Association." *Medical Record News* 49:2 (April 1978): 8–25.

Connell, H. Boyce, Jr. *The Georgia Law of Medical Records.* rev. ed. Atlanta: Georgia Medical Record Association, 1987.

Confidentiality of Alcohol and Drug Abuse Patient Records." *Federal Register,* Department of Health, Education, and Welfare, 1975.

Confidentiality of Alcohol and Drug Abuse Patient Records." *Federal Register,* Department of Health and Human Services, 9 June 1987.

Feste, Laura. "A Position Statement from the American Health Information Management Association: Patient Access to Personal Information." *Journal of AHIMA* 63:3 (March 1992).

_____ . "Practice Bulletin: Guidelines for Faxing Patient Health Information." *Journal of the American Medical Record Association* 62:6 (June 1991): 29–32.

Hadley, Linda. "Risk Management: Confidentiality and Custody." *For The Record* 2:9 (26 February 1990): 1, 4–5, 8–11, 23–24.

Hoyt, Emmanuel. *Medicolegal Aspects of Hospital Records.* Berwyn, Ill.: Physicians' Record Co., 1977.

_____ , Lillian Hoyt, and August Groeschel. *Law of Hospital, Physician, and Patient.* Berwyn, Ill.: Physicians' Record Co., 1972.

Gordes, Leon, and Ellen Gold. "Privacy, Confidentiality, and the Use of Medical Records in Research." *Journal of the American Medical Record Association* 51:6 (December 1980): 24, 105–08.

Hospital Medical Records: Guidelines for Their Use and Release of Medical Information. Chicago: American Hospital Association, 1972.

Huffman, Edna. *Medical Record Management.* Berwyn, Ill.: Physicians' Record Co., 1972.

Jones, Robin. "Of Professional Interest: Medical Record Access Laws." *Journal of AHIMA* 63:3 (March 1992): 29–34.

Management Advisory. *Information Management: Disclosure of Medical Record Information.* Chicago, Ill.: American Hospital Association, 1990.

Manes, Rose. "Patient Rights, Student Rights — Parallel Trends." *Medical Record News* 46:6 (December 1975): 73–76.

Marek, Helen. *Medicolegal Guidelines and Forms for Hospitals.* Corpus Christi, Tex.: Transcription, Inc., 1979.

Southwick, Arthur. *The Law of Hospital and Health Care Administration.* Ann Arbor: University of Michigan, Health Care Administration Press, 1978.

Tomes, Jonathan. *Health Care Records Manual.* Boston, Mass.: Warren Gorham Lamont, 1993.

"Your Health Information Belongs to You," a brochure prepared by the Professional Practice Division, American Health Information Management Association, Chicago, Illinois.

Appendix 1
State Regulations Regarding Health Information

This chart is a report, by state, of medical record statutes. Each state entry lists laws applicable to the topic heading. The topics are medical record issues considered particularly relevant to the statutory requirements for reporting a disease, the laws of disclosure and confidentiality, and the medical record's admissibility as evidence.

Please know that state laws are constantly changing. This chart should be used only as a general guide to the statutes and regulations concerning medical records. Consult the latest state codes and legislative periodicals for changes affecting your state. Also, the list of state AHIMA officers provided in appendix 4 is a good source to consult for the latest information for any given state.

	Abortion	AIDS/HIV	Child Abuse	Confidentialty
Alabama	§26-21-4 to 26-21-7	§§22-11A-1 to 21-11A38	§§30-51-1 to 30-51-11	§27-21A-25 §22-11A-22
Alaska	§08.64.105	§47.20.290	§§47.17.040 to 47.17.060	§§18.23.010 to 18.23.070
Arizona	§36—2153	§32—1457 §36—661 et seq.	§§13—3620 to 13—3620.01	§36—340 §23—908 §32—1855.02 §12—2285
Arkansas	§5-61-101 §20-18-603	§20-15-901 to 20-15-906	§§12-12-506 to 12-12-515	§23-76-129 §25-19-105
California	Pen 11413 Health & S 25955	Health & S 199.30 et seq. CC 56.28 Health & S 199.215 Health & S 199.27, 199.98 Health & S 199.42 et seq.	Pen 11166, 11167 Pen 851.7	CC 56 et seq.
Colorado	§18-6-101	§25-4-1402.5 §25-4-1405 §25-4-1404	§19-3-308 §19-1-120 §19-1-102	§25-1-107 §25-1-122 §25-1-801
Connecticut	§19a-601(a) to 19a-601(e)	§19a-583(a) §§19a-585(b) to 19a-585(d)	§§17a-101(g) to 17a-101(h)	§52-1466 §19a-215 §20-7c(b)
Delaware	Tit. 24, §1794	Tit. 16, §§1206A to 1207A Tit. 16, §§1202 to 1203	Tit. 31, §3609 Tit. 16, §904	Tit. 24, §1768
District of Columbia	§22-201	§6-2805 §35-226	§6-2113 §§6-2126 to 6-2127	§§32-501 to 32-505
Florida	§390.002 §406.11	§381.004 §§384.25 to 384.27 §760.50 §641.3007 §455.2416	§§415.51 to 415.513 §§415.502 to 415.507	§455.241 §458.339 §405.01 et seq. §409.910 §743.0645

Mental Health	Sexual Offenses	Substance Abuse	Notes
§§22-50-60 to 22-50-62	§15-1-2 §§15-20-3 to 15-20-5	§20-2-56	
§§47.30.845 to 47.30.850	§12.62.035 §§18.66.010 to 18.66.900	§47.37.220	
§§36—517.01 to 36—517.02 §36—509 §36—568.01	§13—3823 §13—1414	§36—2003 §§36—2028 to 36—2029 §13—3412	
§§20-46-103 to 20-46-104	§16-42-101	§20-64-812	
Pen 1543 et seq. Welf & I 5540 et seq. Welf & I 5328 Welf & I 5325	Pen 1620 Pen 13516	Welf & I 5328.15 Health & S 1795.18 CC 56.30	
§27-10-120 §27-10-120.5	§18-3-415 §18-3-410 §13-25-131	§16-11.5-103 §§25-1-209 to 25-1-210 §25-1-1108 §12-22-320	
§17a-548 §§17a-498(b) to 17a-499	§52-146k	§17a-630	
Tit. 16, §§5006 to 5011	Tit. 11, §§3508 to 3509	Tit. 16, §2214 Tit. 16, 2204	
§§6-2011 to 6-2015 §6-2051	§22-3506	§24-524	
§394.459 §394.907	§943.325 §905.035 §951.27 §960.003	§953.15 §440.102 §397.057	

	Abortion	AIDS/HIV	Child Abuse	Confidentialty
Georgia	§15-11-114	§§24-9-40.1 to 24-9-47 §31-22-9.1 to 31-22-9.2	§19-7-5 §§49-5-40 to 49-5-46	§§24-9-41 to 24-9-45 §31-33-6
Hawaii	§453-16 §18-604	§§325-101 to 325-104	§350-1.4 §587-81	§92F-14 §622-57 §325-4 §324-32
Idaho	§§18-604 to 18-612 §54-1814	§§39-609 to 39-610	§32-717A	§§39-1392 to 39-1392e §54-1820 §39-1394
Illinois	§720 ILCS 510/11[38 81-31] §720 ILCS 510/10	§410 ILCS 305/1 et seq. §410 ILCS 305/9 [111½] §410 ILCS 305/9 [111½ 7309]	§325 ILCS 5/5 §325 ILCS 5/10 §325 ILCS 5/11 §20 ILCS 510/65.8	§410 ILCS 325/8 §410 ILCS 50/3 [111½ 5403]
Indiana	§35-1-58.5-5	§16-1-9.5-2 §16-1-10.5-11.5	§31-6-11-18 §31-6-8-1	§16-4-8-1 to 16-4-8-14
Iowa	§331.802 §707.7 et seq.	§141.23-141.24 §141.10	§232.74 §232.69 et seq.	§217.30 §147A.10 §22.7 §135.42
Kansas	§65-445	§§65-6001 et seq.	§65-525 §65-512 §§38-122 to 38-123b	§40-4407 §45-221 §65-102b §65-118
Kentucky	Self-Consent Rule A	§§214.181, 214.625 §§214.400 to 214.420 §311.282	§§15.900 to 15.940	§§422.315 to 422.330 §311.591 §§214.400 to 214.420
Louisiana	§40:1299.35.10	§37:1747 §40:1300.11 et seq. §40:12.99.40 §40:1299.142	§46.56 §14:403 §ChC 609 et seq.	§22:2020 §40:2017.9 §40:1299.87 §40:1299.96 §44:7
Maine	Tit. 22 § 1596	Tit. 5 § 19203 et seq. Tit. 22 § 1711-B	Tit. 22 § 4016 Tit. 15 § 321	Tit. 22 § 3291 Tit. 9-B § 161 Tit. 5 § 200-E

Mental Health	Sexual Offenses	Substance Abuse	Notes
§§37-3-166 to 37-3-168 §37-1-53	§16-6-23 §24-2-3 §24-4-62	§37-7-166 §26-5-17 §37-8-50	
§334-5 §334E-2	§§707-730 to 707-733	§§334-121 to 334-134 §329-54	
§66-348	§18-6105	§37-2743 §37-3102	
§5 ILCS 160/7 §740 ILCS 110/5 §740 ILCS 110/6	§215 ILCS 5/356e §215 ILCS 125/4-4 §730 ILCS 5/5-3-4	§720 ILCS 570/406	
§16-4-8-3.2 §16-4-8-3.1	§35-37-44	§§12-23-1-1 to 12-23-17-3	
§229.25 §622.10 §135H.11	§22.7 §709.15	§125.37 §125.33	
§65-5601 et seq. §76-12b11	§22-3426 §§75-5218 to 75-5220	§65-657 §65-4121	
§202B.180 §202B.990	§17.160 §510.300	§§222.70 to 222.80 §210.670	
§37:1114 §§ChC 1416 to 1417 §§CE 510 §ChC 1453	§15:579 §40:2109.1	§37:3384	
Tit. 34-B § 1205 Tit. 34-B § 1207	Tit. 16 § 53-A	Tit. 32 § 7004 Tit. 22 § 3173-D	

	Abortion	AIDS/HIV	Child Abuse	Confidentialty
Maryland	§20-103	HG §18-336 to §18-338.1 HG §18-207 HG §18-213	FL §5-704 to 5-711	HG §4-302 HG §4-401
Massachusetts	§29:20B §112:12Q	§111:2F §70F	§§119:51A to 119:51F §112:12F §118E:1A, 6B, 15	§1751:2 §112:12CC
Michigan	§25.248(104) MCR §5.783	§14.15(5114-5114a) §14.15(5117) §14.15(5121) §14.15(5133) §14.15(2843b)	§25.248(3) §25.248(6) §25.248(13)	MCR §2.314(D)-(f)
Minnesota	§145.413	§214.19 §72A.20 §611A.19 §114.768	§§626.561 to 626.562 §626.556	§144.335 §148B.64 et seq.
Mississippi	§§41-41-55 to 41-41-61	§41-41-16 §99-19-201	§§44-24-3 to 43-24-5 §43-19-45	§43-13-121 §13-1-21 §41-9-67 §41-9-107
Missouri	§188.110 §188.210	§191.656	§337.636 §337.639	§208.155 §109.280
Montana	§50-20-110 §50-20-105	§50-16-1003 §50-16-1007 §50-16-1009 §50-16-1013	§41-3-205 §52-2-203 §52-2-211	§33-31-113 §50-16-525 §50-16-602 §50-16-205
Nebraska	§28-330 et seq. §28-336 §28-345	§20-167	§28-719 §§28-725 to 28-726	§68-1025
Nevada	§442.256 §422.265	§441A.320	§§432B.280 to 432B.290 §432.120	§449.650 §629.061
New Hampshire	§§141-F:7 to 141-F:8	§§141-F:7 to 141-F:11	§169-C:25 §169-C:35	§329:26 §151:21 §332-I:1

Mental Health	Sexual Offenses	Substance Abuse	Notes
HG §4-307 HG §10-713 CJ §5-316	27, §461A HG §15-127	HG §17-214.1 HG §8-205	
§19:16 §112:129A §123:23 §36A	§112:12A1/2 §265:24C	§111B §123:36A §11E:14	
§14.800(141) §14.800(143a) §14.800(723) §14.800(746-750) §14.800(946)	§27A.2157(1)	§14.15(6111) §14.15(6124) §14.15(6521)	
§148B.66 §245.696 §253C.01 §253B.12	§244.05 §609.1351	§595.02 §609.3452 §243.16 §243.166	
§41-21-102 §§41-21-7 to 41-21-13 §41-21-97	§§45-31-7 to 45-31-9 §§97-3-65 to 97-3-73	§71-7-3 §71-7-5	
§630.080	§191.225	§208.152	
§§53-21-141 to 53-21-142 §50-16-535	§§46-18-254 to 46-18-255 §§46-23-501 to 46-23-507	§41-1-403 §53-24-302 §53-24-306	
§83-1068 §§20-161 to 20-166	§81-1842	§71-5030	
§433A.360 §§433A.701 to 433A.711 §433.332	§44.069 §50.090	§458.280 §453.720	
§135-C:19-a	§632-A:17	§318-B:12-a §172:8-a	

	Abortion	AIDS/HIV	Child Abuse	Confidentialty
New Jersey	§26:5C-5 §26:6-8.2 et seq.	§26:5C-5 et seq. §26:6-8.2 et seq.	§9:6-8, 10a §9:6-8:47	17B:21-5
New Mexico	§24-14-18	§§24-2B-1 to 24-2B-6	§§32-1-44 to 32-1-45	§14-3A-2 §14-6-1 §24-1-20
New York	PUB HE §17	PUB HE §§2780 to 2782	SOC S §422	CPLR §3101 PUB HE §17
North Carolina	§14-46 §14-45.1, (c)	§130A-143	§§7A-543 to 7A-549	§131E-213 §143-578 §8-44.1
North Dakota	§14-02.1-03.3 §14-02.1-07	§23-07-02.2 §23-07.5-05	§§50-25.1-03 to 1-07 §50-25.1-14	§23-01-12 §44-04-18.1 §23-17.1-06
Ohio	§2317.56	§§3701.24.2 to 3701.24.3	§§2151.14 to 2151.14.1	§2953.35 §3701.74
Oklahoma	Tit. 63 §§1-736 to 1-739 Tit. 59§524	Tit. 63 §§1-502.2 to 1-502.3	Tit. 22 §753 Tit. 10 §1125.2 Tit. 21 §§846 to 848	Tit. 43A §1-109 Tit. 56 §1004 Tit. 76 §19
Oregon	§432.005 §432.120	§433.060 et seq. §433.075	§418.770 §418.990	§192.525 §192.530 §441.750
Pennsylvania	Tit. 18 Pa. C.S.A. §3214	Tit. 35 P.S. §7601 et seq.	Tit. 23 Pa. C.S.A. §6335 Tit. 23 Pa. C.S.A. §6381	Tit. 23 Pa. C.S.A. §5309 Tit. 42 Pa. C.S.A. §6159 Tit. 42 Pa. C.S.A. §5929
Rhode Island	Const. R.I., Art. I, §2	§§23-6-17 to 23-6-20	§23-51-1 §40-11-13	§5-37-22 §5-37.3-4 §9-19-27 §38-2-2

Mental Health	Sexual Offenses	Substance Abuse	Notes
§30:4-24.3 §26:8-5 §30:4-126.1	§2C:25-16 §2C:25-28	§26:2B-15 §26:2L-4 §9:17A-4	
§43-1-19	§29-11-6 §30-9-16	§26-2-12 §26-2-14	
CPL §730.20 MENT HY §81.09	CIV R §50-c	MENT HY §19.07	
§§122C-52 to 122C-55	§143B-480.2, (c) 8C-1, Rule 412	§90-109.1, (a)	
§25-03.1-43 to 25-03.1-45	§12.1-20-07	§25-03.1-43 to 25-03.1-45	
§5119.43	§2907.02 §2907.11	§3335.15.1	
Tit. 43A §1-109 Tit. 43A §2-301 Tit. 43A §2-208	Tit. 51 §24A.8 Tit. 57 §584	Tit. 43A §§3-422 to 3-423	
§426.175	§147.115	§430.345 §430.405	
Tit. 50 P.S. §4605 Tit. 50 P.S. §7111 Tit. 50 P.S. §7108	Tit. 42 Pa. C.S.A. §5945.1	Tit. 71 P.S. §1690.104 Tit. 71 P.S. §1690.108	
§40.1-5.3-15 §40.1-21-9	§11-37-13 Super. Ct. Crim. Rule 26.3	§21-28.2-4 §21-28.3-3	

	Abortion	AIDS/HIV	Child Abuse	Confidentialty
South Carolina	§44-41-60 §44-41-34	§44-29-80 §44-29-90 §44-29-135 §44-29-146	§20-7-690 §20-7-520 §20-7-560 §20-7-650	§8-11-110
South Dakota	§34-23A-10 §34-23A-19	§34-23-2	§26-8a-11 §26-8a-13 §26-8a-15	§58-4-45 §58-41-73
Tennessee	§39-15-203	§68-5-102 §68-10-113	§37-1-612	§68-6-219 §10-7-504 §68-11-304 §63-6-219
Texas	H&S §245.011	H&S §§81.103 to 81.109	Fam §34.011 Fam §34.04 Fam §34.08 Fam §35.01	Civ. Stat. 4495b §5.08
Utah	§26-18-4 §76-7-302 §76-7-313	§26-6-3 §64-13-36	§62A-4-506 §62A-4-513	§21-1-17.5 §78-25-25
Vermont	Tit. 12 §1705 Tit. 18 §1128	Tit. 12 §1705	Tit. 33 §§4916 to 4919	Tit. 26 §1443
Virginia	§32.1-264	§§32.1-36 to 32.1-45.2	§16.1-300	§2.1-342 §§42.1-77 to 42.1-79.1 §16.1-88.2 §8.01-413 §8.01-399
Washington	§43.70.160	§70.24.320 et seq. §70.24.015 §70.24.022 §70.24.105	§26.44.030 §5.60.060 §26.44.035	§70.02.020 et seq.
West Virginia	§16-2F-4 §16-2F-6	§16-29-1 §§16-3C-1 to 16-3C-9	§§49-6B-1 to 49-6B-4 §49-7-1 §49-7-23	§5A-8-13 §33-25A-26 §§57-5-4a to 57-5-4j
Wisconsin	§48.375 §48.396 §895.037	§146.022 §146.025	§48.981	§146.81 et seq.

Mental Health	Sexual Offenses	Substance Abuse	Notes
§44-22-110 §44-22-120 §44-23-1100 §44-26-120	§16-3-730	§44-9-10 §8-11-110	
§§27a-12-25 to 27A-12-32	§§23A-22-15 to 23A-22-15.1	§34-20A-90 §23-5-10 §36-4-22.1	
§33-3-104	Evid. Rule 412 §39-13-521	§33-8-508 §10-7-504	
H&S §595.001 et seq. H&S §611.001 et seq. H&S §576.005	Civ. Stat. §4413(51) CCrP §57.01 et seq.	H&S §462.003 H&S §462.064	
§62A-12-247	§§78-3c-1 to 78-3c-4 §77-27-21.5	§34-38-13	
Tit. 3 §206	Tit. 13 §3253 Tit. 13 §3255 Tit. 13 §5301	Tit. 6 §1165	
§2.1-342	§18.2-67.7	§54.1-3406	
§26.44.060	§70.125.065 §§4.24.550 to 4.24.555	§66.16.090 §69.50.410	
§27-3-1	§61-8B-13	§16-1-10	
§51.30 §905.04 §51.61	§146.82 §940.225	§51.45 §51.30	

	Abortion	AIDS/HIV	Child Abuse	Confidentialty
Wyoming	§35-6-108	§35-4-132	§14-3-210	§§35-2-601 to 35-2-617

Mental Health	Sexual Offenses	Substance Abuse	Notes
§25-10-122	§6-2-312	§§33-38-101 to 33-38-110	

Appendix 2
Developing a Confidentiality Policy

Any healthcare facility or practice that might have occasion to release information in response to requests from third parties is well advised to develop its own confidentiality policy. Such a policy acts as a further safeguard against the possibility of unwanted and potentially costly litigation resulting from a breach of patient confidentiality by providing those charged with the responsibility for releasing information with confidentiality guidelines specific to the mission and needs of the facility or practice.

As with any undertaking, preparation is the most important ingredient and is the key to ensuring the development of a policy custom-tailored to your provider's needs. Prior to writing the policy, familiarize yourself with the applicable state and federal laws and regulations and ascertain the needs of your facility or practice relative to the release of information. Sources to check include but are not limited to state health general, confidentiality, record retention, and mandatory reporting laws, and the Federal Register.

Know the Law

Obtaining a working knowledge of relevant laws and regulations frequently entails an analysis of the same — some of which may appear to conflict — to determine which take precedence in different situations. Although the law that most strictly protects a patient's right to privacy usually takes precedence, there are times when a statute or regulation may contain a statement to the contrary. The best advice here is to compare the statutes carefully.

In developing your policy, consider the legal requirements as the minimum standard. It is important to recognize that the law is not all inclusive; it could never hope to cover all the possible situations that might arise. It is wise and much more useful to users of the policy to go beyond the law in protecting patient confidentiality. When this is done, however, be sure it is clearly indicated in your policy statement.

Ascertain Your Specific Needs

Keeping in mind that your confidentiality policy is really the application of the law to the information practices and needs of your facility or practice, you will be making informed choices about how to handle specific situations within the parameters of the law. In order to be able to do this, thoroughly research the following:

- ▸ Your facility's operational and organizational plans
- ▸ How information is stored and maintained
- ▸ To whom and why most information is released
- ▸ The patient's right of access to his or her own records
- ▸ Problems that may arise and how to deal with them

What to Include in a Confidentiality Policy

There are several sections that should be included and topics that must be addressed in your confidentiality policy. Consider the items listed below and fine tune them to your particular needs.

Introduction to the Policy

Include in the Introduction a general statement that outlines the philosophy and mission of your facility or practice as well as a statement to the effect that, although the physical patient records are the property of the provider, the information contained therein belongs to the patients and may be utilized on their behalf. Stress the goal of protecting a patient's right to confidentiality as well as the interests of the facility or provider.

This section should also include an itemization of the laws and regulations that specifically address your needs and information practices. This itemization should be accompanied by a glossary of terms that appear in those laws or that clarify the provisions of your policy.

General Information Practices

This section specifies how certain situations are to be handled. In developing this section you will have to make some basic policy decisions because not all issues encountered in the day-to-day handling of information are addressed by law. Some specific issues that must be addressed include:

- ▸ The scope of information covered by disclosure requirements, including oral and written communications and requests for information

- ▸ The handling of information pertaining to family members of the patient of record so that consideration is extended to all who may be a subject of information released

- ▸ Whether or not to include a statement prohibiting redisclosure with all written information released and the specific wording to be used

- ▸ How to handle information/records received from other facilities or providers. Do you release the information with the proper consent or do you route the requester back to the facility that generated the information?

- ▸ Whether or not all requests for information must be in writing

- ▸ A record of disclosures (what information was released and to whom) is documented in a release of information log as well as in the individual patient record

- ▸ The designation of a custodian of the records and a description of how the records are physically secured

- ▸ Communication of the policy's provisions to employees, students, volunteers, and patients via distribution of the written policy, in-service training, brochures, etc.

Patient Authorizations

This section must include what constitutes a valid consent and define who, legally, has the authority to authorize the release of information in any given situation. It is important to identify who may authorize disclosures if the patient is a minor, is legally incompetent, is in need of mental health treatment but has not been adjudged incompetent by a court, or is deceased.

Disclosures without Patient Authorization

This section discusses the situations where, according to statute or regulation, information can or must be released without the patient's authorization. Decide if you want to use all the exceptions allowed by permissive/voluntary disclosure laws. Also identify those cases where mandatory reporting is required, such as child abuse reporting. Be sure that the policy specifies in what cases and to whom information may be released. Laws are usually very specific in the area of mandatory/voluntary reporting — your policy should reflect that.

Patient Access

The patient access section spells out whether or not patients have a legal right of access to their records and, in the absence of such a right whether or not the provider will extend the privilege of inspecting and/or obtaining photocopies of their records to the patients. Specify any cases where this privilege would be restricted, such as minors or legally incompetent patients.

Reasonable Fees

Define the fees that your provider charges a requester for photocopies of records, abstracts, or record searches. Keep in mind that professional courtesy dictates that healthcare providers are never charged for medical information for continuity of care.

Your policy should also state whether or not patients are allowed, by statute or provider privilege, to correct and/or amend inaccurate information in their records. If this is allowed, spell out the procedure to be followed.

Penalties for Negligence

It is not only wise to know the penalties for negligence in releasing information; the penalties — be they criminal, civil, or organizational sanctions — should be clearly stated in your policy. Also, if your facility or provider gives recourse to patients via a grievance procedure, the procedure should be set forth in the policy.

Forms

To round out your policy, attach a set of forms used in the release of medical information process such as your general authorization to release medical information form, fax transmission sheet, additional information form, abstracts, or consent to film or tape a patient care encounter.

A sample of a release of information policy follows, and appendix 5 contains forms for your use and review. Consult the alphabetized topics portion of this guide for more specific information relevant to those issues discussed here.

Sample Release of Information Policy

This is only a partial outline of a release of information policy to serve as a guide to get you started. (Statements in parentheses are to be completed by the individual facility.)

Policy

Direct all requests for release of information received by the facility to the Medical Record Department for processing.

All information in patient records shall be kept confidential and secure. Release of information from patient records complies with federal, state and local laws.

Patient records are the property of the facility and may be removed only in accordance with a court order or subpoena. Access is limited to authorized personnel.

Subpoenas served in person or received through the mail are processed by the correspondence copy service, which delivers the chart to the court or sends copies to attorneys.

Requests for copies of patient records are processed by the correspondence clerk. A correspondence copying service copies the requested records, mails them, and bills for this service.

Records are kept on file as original hard copy for four years and are then microfilmed.

Patient records will be available for use within the facility for patient care by all authorized personnel as documented in a policy manual specified by the chief executive officer.

Confidential information may be released with specific and informed authorization as described below:

Authorizations

(Include sample general authorization)

The authorization is valid if it contains the following information:

1. Name of facility that is to release information.
2. Name of person or institution and address to whom the information is to be given.
3. Name of the patient, patient address, date of birth, and/or social security number.
4. Purpose for the disclosure.
5. Specific time period to be covered and the extent or nature of information to be released.
6. Signature of the patient or legal representative.
7. Dated at time of signature (void after ____ days).
8. Date of authorization that does not retroactively release information.

The authorization shall be filed in the patient record with a notation of what information was released, the date it was released, and who released it.

The patient may revoke a prior authorization at any time in writing.

Refusal to Honor Authorization

The facility will refuse to honor a written authorization if there is:

1. Reasonable doubt as to the identity of the person presenting the authorization, or evidence that the person requesting the information is not the person named in the authorization.
2. Evidence that the patient is not legally authorized to disclose the information or if there is a serious question regarding the patient's mental capacity to understand what they have authorized by their signature.
3. Evidence that the person signing for a minor or incompetent person is not legally qualified to do so.
4. Reason to suspect the patient's signature is not authentic.
5. Reason to question the current validity of an authorization because it appears to be a perpetual release with no time limits set.
6. Evidence allowing release before the service is rendered.

7. Evidence in the patient record of sensitive information that cannot be released to third-party payers using the blanket Conditions of Admission authorization.

Patient Access

(Patient access laws vary in each state, so include the policy according to your location. Specify age limitations and how to handle special sensitive information).

Minors

The authorization must be signed by a parent or legal guardian if the patient is under (specify age limits according to your state and local laws).

Not all minors require the consent of their parent or guardian. (Specify here all the details and conditions under which minors may consent on their own according to your state and local laws).

After Death

If a patient has died, authorization disclosing information in the decedent's patient record must be signed by the administrator or executor of the decedent's estate. If there is no probate administrator, authorization can be signed by the surviving spouse or next of kin.

Telephone Requests

In emergency situations, it may be in the patient's best interest to release information by telephone to a physician who is currently treating the patient. Inform the caller that the information will be retrieved and the call will be returned. Using the telephone directory or physician's list, check the telephone number of the caller. Release only the minimum amount of information by telephone.

Physicians (Not on the Medical Staff) and Other Healthcare Facilities

A written authorization from the patient is required prior to filling requests for information. In emergency situations, information can be given over the telephone.

Employers

A written authorization from the patient is required.

Attorneys

A written authorization from the patient is required.

Law Enforcement Officials

A written authorization from the patient, a court order, or subpoena is required. (Reference your state and local laws for blood alcohol test results obtained through the Emergency Department.)

Research and Education

Studies requiring review of selected patient records by members of the hospital's medical staff do not need the patient's authorization, provided the identity of each patient is not revealed. Requests for research and educational studies from outside the medical staff need approval from the Medical Staff Executive Committee. Use of any information identifying the patient requires the patient's written authorization.

Blue Cross and Other Third-Party Payers for Claims Processing

Authorizations are not required for releasing information for payers of the bill, except for selected sensitive information for which a special authorization is required (be specific here as to the sensitive information—drug and alcohol abuse, child and elder abuse, HIV test results, or psychiatric care). Conditions of admission authorizations should have a statement covering release of this information.

News Media

Refer to Public Relations or Administration.

Government Agencies

The facility department with the reporting responsibility should be listed here. Examples to be included in this section:

1. No-fault automobile insurance laws may or may not require patient authorizations, but they may require reporting to an insurance carrier and permit copies of records to be sent to the carrier. (Emergency Department)

2. Communicable disease laws usually require reporting without patient authorization. (Infection Control)

3. Cancer reporting and registry laws usually require reporting to a state agency without patient authorization. (Medical Records)

4. Criminally inflicted injuries usually require reporting to local police departments without patient authorization. (Emergency Department and Medical Staff)

5. Child and elder protective service laws usually require reporting to a state agency without patient authorization. (Emergency Room and Medical Staff)

Mental Health Records (Psychiatric)

Laws relevant to psychiatric patient records vary a great deal from state to state, so no attempt has been made here to provide sample policy statements. Provide here a copy of your laws, and a sample of the special authorization, if a special authorization is needed, and the conditions under which information may be released without a patient authorization not only pursuant to subpoenas and court orders, but to patients, third party payers, government agencies, and other requesters.

Substance Abuse Records

Although there is a federal law governing these records, many states and local governments have more restrictive laws that override the federal regulations, therefore the same type of information should be added here as is mentioned in the Mental Health Records section.

Adapted with permission from Vicki Carlisle, "Alternative Staffing Services: Correspondence Copiers," *Journal of AHIMA* 63, No. 3 (March 1992): 56–57.

Appendix 3
AHIMA Position Statement: Patient Access to Personal Health Information

Summary of the Issue

The health record is the physical property of the healthcare provider who compiles, stores, and maintains the data. Providers must keep records to document the services they render. This information may be released only with written authorization from the patient, the patient's legal representative, or as granted by law. The information in health records is routinely used by third parties such as employers, insurers, and other healthcare providers as the basis for making decisions that affect the patient. Yet patients are not routinely granted access to their health information.

Laws regulating patient access to health records are not uniform or even universal. Federal regulations for substance abuse programs, 42 CFR Part 2, "Confidentiality of Alcohol and Drug Abuse Patient Records," specifically permit individuals access to their own health records. Subpart B, Section 2.23 states: "These regulations do not prohibit a program from giving a patient access to his or her own records, including the opportunity to inspect and copy any records that the program maintains about the patient." Section 483.10(b)(2) of the new OBRA regulations for nursing facilities grants residents access to their records within 24 hours, and grants residents the right to obtain photocopies within two working days. Only 27 states have statutes requiring providers to make health records available to patients, and the majority of these statutes fall under hospital licensing acts. Because of the absence of these regulations, individuals are routinely denied access to their health information.

AHIMA's Position

The American Health Information Management Association believes that patients should have access to the information contained in their health records. Patients have the right to access their health records so they can:

▸ Be knowledgeable about the nature of their disease or health status and understand the treatment and prognosis.

▸ Be educated about their health status to enable them to participate actively in their treatment process and in wellness programs.

▸ Provide a history of their medical care to a new healthcare provider.

▸ Ensure the accuracy of documentation in the health record with regards to diagnoses, treatment(s), and their response to treatment(s).

▸ Verify that the documentation in the health record supports the provider's bill for services.

▸ Be informed of the nature of the information being released to third parties, such as insurers, when authorizing disclosure of their health information.

AHIMA's Recommendations

Patients or their representatives may have access to their own health records upon presentation of a properly completed and signed authorization, with reasonable notice, except:

▸ Where state law specifically precludes access

▸ Minors governed by legal constraints

▸ Patients adjudicated as incompetent

▸ Situations where the healthcare provider has determined information would be injurious to patient or other persons

Patients should not bear unreasonable charges for obtaining copies of health records. But patients and their representatives must also acknowledge that the provider is entitled to charges that are sufficient to cover all reasonable costs associated with providing patient access to health records.*

If the patient's request is denied the provider must:

▸ Provide a summary in a reasonable time

▸ Permit inspection by or provide copies of the health records to another healthcare practitioner who has been so designated, in writing, by the patient or legal representative

▸ Include with the health record a statement from the healthcare provider explaining the reason for refusal

The health record is the permanent, legal document that must contain sufficient information to identify the patient and describe the diagnosis and treatment. In order for the health records to provide the information individuals need to take an active role in their healthcare and maintenance, the following guidelines should be followed to ensure accurate and complete information in both computer-based and paper health records:

- ▸ An individual health record is established for each person receiving care
- ▸ All individual patient health data are properly identified by patient name and a unique personal identifier
- ▸ Clinical data, including history and physical, and results of diagnostic tests that support the diagnosis, are maintained in the health record
- ▸ Clinical data are recorded at the time service is provided and reflect the encounter date
- ▸ Treatment plans reflect plan of action, frequency of therapy, duration, and dosage of medications
- ▸ Clinical assessments form a chronological picture of the course of a patient's health status and include test results, follow-up, and response to treatment
- ▸ A standard set of data is collected for every patient
- ▸ All entries must include title of author, date (month, day, year), and authentication either by written signature, initials, or electronic signature
- ▸ Handwritten entries in a paper health record must be legible and recorded in ink or typewritten
- ▸ Abbreviations and symbols used in the health record must be clearly defined
- ▸ Corrections to the health record must be made as an addendum, without change or deletion to the original entry. The addendum should be identified as such and include the date and time of the correction, and the identity of the person making the correction.
- ▸ Patient corrections to the health record are treated as an addendum to the original entry, without changing the original. The addendum should be clearly identified as such and added to the health record at the direction of the patient.

Conclusion

AHIMA believes the health record is the physical property of the healthcare provider who compiles, stores, and maintains the data. However, the information in the health record belongs to the patient. AHIMA promotes patient access to their health records in order to empower them to take an active role in decisions regarding their personal lives based on the information in their health records.

Prepared by Laura K. Feste, RRA, assistant director, Professional Practice Division

Approved by the AHIMA Board of Directors January 1992

* Lou Ann Schraffendberger, R.R.A., "Of Professional Interest: Contracting with Photocopy Services," *Journal of AHIMA* 63, No. 1 (March 1992): 25.

Appendix 4
State AHIMA
Officers

Please note that this list was the most current available when compilation of this book was completed. As with most associations of national scope, its state officers can change yearly. The date after the individual's name is the month his or her term expires in 1995, and the telephone number is the business number.

Alabama
Julie Marshall, R.R.A. (May)
Health Information Department
Thomas Hospital
P.O. Drawer 929
Fairhope, AL 36533
(205) 928-2375

Alaska
Charlene R. Thompson, A.R.T. (May)
Our Lady of Compassion Care Center
HC01 Box 6201 AB
Palmer, AK 99645
(907) 762-0273

Arizona
Patricia Nelson, A.R.T. (April)
2601 W. Winchomb
Phoenix, AZ 85023
(602) 863-0943

Arkansas
Linda Bottoms Feltner, A.R.T. (May)
9708 Croxted
Fort Smith, AR 72903
(501) 441-4054

California
Cynthia M. Doyon, R.R.A. (May)
Hospital Correspondence Corp.
688 N. Rimsdale Avenue, #99
Covina, CA 91722
(310) 949-9811

Colorado
LeAnn Blackmon, R.R.A. (May)
Colorado Mental Health Institute
1600 W. 24th Street
Pueblo, CO 81003
(719) 546-4221

Connecticut

Mary Jane Cook, R.R.A. (June)

Lawrence and Memorial Hospital

365 Montauk Avenue

New London, CT 06320

(203) 442-0711 ext. 2625

Delaware

Marybeth Besosa, R.R.A. (June)

20 Rawlings Drive

Bear, DE 19701

(302) 651-4462

District of Columbia

Margaret M. Elliott, A.R.T. (June)

7045 Leebrad Street

Springfield, VA 22151

(202) 293-6554

Florida

Perry Ellie, R.R.A. (June)

9242 123 Avenue North

Largo, FL 34643

(813) 586-6989

Georgia

Art Bell, R.R.A. (Sept.)

130 Loblolly Road

Moultrie, GA 31768

(912) 890-3439

Hawaii

Miki K. Masuda, R.R.A. (Aug.)

Director of Medical Records

Shriner's Hospital for Crippled Children

1310 Punahou

Honolulu, HI 96826

(808) 941-4466

Idaho

Deanna Schmidt, A.R.T. (May)

2700 Beverly

Boise, ID 83709

(208) 378-2388

Illinois

Lou Ann Schraffenberger, R.R.A. (April)

University of Illinois at Chicago

Department of Health Information Management (M/C 520)

1919 W. Taylor Street, Room 811

Chicago, IL 60612

(312) 996-3530

Indiana

Kathy Grider, R.R.A. (April)

P.O. Box 284

Pendleton, IN 46038

(317) 778-2080

Iowa

Sandra Peters, A.R.T. (May)

Mercy Hospital

500 East Market Street

Iowa City, IA 52245

(319) 339-3829

Kansas
Joe D. Gillespie, R.R.A. (Sept.)
St. Francis Regional Medical Center
929 N. St. Francis
Wichita, KS 67214
(316) 268-5850

Kentucky
Jennie L. Bryan, R.R.A. (May)
706 Quails Run Boulevard
Louisville, KY 40207
(800) 264-5080

Louisiana
Anita Hazelwood, R.R.A. (March)
P.O. Box 41007 USL
Lafayette, LA 70504
(318) 231-6633

Maine
Nancy E. Tracy, A.R.T. (June)
Acadia Hospital, P.O. Box 391
Brewer, ME 04412
(207) 990-6139

Maryland
Patricia Brown, R.R.A. (March)
1563 Andover Lane
Frederick, MD 21702
(301) 790-8131

Massachusetts
Louise G. Corcoran, A.R.T. (June)
Director, Medical Records
Holyoke Hospital, Inc.
575 Beech Street
Holyoke, MA 01040
(413) 534-2567

Michigan
Pat Rublo, R.R.A. (May)
Schoolcraft College
1751 Radcliffe
Garden City, MI 48135
(313) 462-4770

Minnesota
Kathleen Swensen, A.R.T. (Sept.)
Rice Memorial Hospital
301 Becker Avenue SW
Willmar, MN 56201
(612) 231-4681

Mississippi
Martha Lawrence, A.R.T. (June)
P.O. Box 677
Kosciusko, MS 39090
(601) 289-4311

Missouri
Cathy Cole, R.R.A. (Sept.)
St. John's Regional Medical Center
2727 McClelland Boulevard
Joplin, MO 64804
(417) 625-2171

Montana
Billie Holmlund, R.R.A. (April and Oct.)
3902 Lost Creek Road, Apt. 3
Anaconda, MT 59711
(406) 563-8500

Nebraska
Cindy M. Smith, A.R.T. (Sept.)
2717 Butterfoot Lane
Hastings, NE 68901
(402) 461-5174

Nevada
Chris Thorne, R.R.A. (April)
2140 Burnside Drive
Sparks, NV 89431
(702) 328-4362

New Hampshire
Carolyn Brennan, A.R.T. (June)
New Hampshire Hospital
105 Pleasant Street
Concord, NH 03301
(603) 271-5520

New Jersey
Laureen Rimmer, R.R.A. (June)
St. Francis Medical Center
601 Hamilton Avenue
Trenton, NJ 08629
(609) 599-5205

New Mexico
Melody Brashear, A.R.T. (May)
3408 Chee Dodge
Gallup, NM 87301
(505) 863-7055

New York
Elizabeth Wheeler, R.R.A. (June)
Health Care Plan
130 Empire Drive
West Seneca, NY 14224
(716) 668-6170

North Carolina
Susan Thomason, R.R.A. (May)
120-B Kingston Drive
Chapel Hill, NC 27514
(919) 944-7188

North Dakota
Nanci Schwindt, R.R.A. (May)
MedCenter One
300 North 7th Street
Bismarck, ND 58501
(701) 224-6160

Ohio
Debbie Schrubb, R.R.A. (April)
Good Samaritan Hospital
2222 Philadelphia Drive
Dayton, OH 45406
(513) 278-2612 ext. 1425

Oklahoma
Verna C. McNabb, R.R.A. (Sept.)
512 Sunburst Street
Norman, OK 73069
(405) 360-8362

Oregon
Diane Davis, R.R.A. (March)
Sisters of Providence Health Plans in Oregon
Utilization and Quality Management
1235 N.E. 47th, Suite 220
Portland, OR 97213
(503) 280-7614

Pennsylvania
Janet Anderson, R.R.A. (May)
Geisinger Medical Center
100 N. Academy Avenue
Danville, PA 17822
(717) 271-8173

Puerto Rico
Gertrudys Nieves-Burrero, R.R.A. (Sept.)
Urb. Vista Azul
Calle 22 S-2
Arecibo, PR 00612
(809) 878-7272

Rhode Island
Jean Beando, R.R.A. (May)
1650 Douglas Avenue, Apt. 3210
North Providence, RI 02904
(401) 456-3091

South Carolina
Susan J. McCammon, R.R.A. (July)
Health South Rehabilitation
2935 Colonial Drive
Columbia, SC 29203
(803) 254-7777 ext. 156

South Dakota
Joelyn M. Sherley, R.R.A. (Sept.)
303 North 4th Street, #4
Aberdeen, SD 57401
(605) 622-5192

Tennessee
Fredia H. Hall, R.R.A. (Nov.)
Centennial Medical Center
230 25th Avenue North
Nashville, TN 37203
(615) 342-3888

Texas
Pamela R. Yokubaitis, R.R.A. (Aug.)
17414 Fountainview Circle
Sugarland, TX 77479
(713) 436-1867

Utah
Patti Slaughter, A.R.T. (March)
Davis Hospital and Medical Center
1600 W. Antelope Drive
Layton, UT 84041
(801) 774-7115

Vermont
Carol Stocker, R.R.A. (Sept. – every 2 yrs.)
28 Winding Brook Drive
South Burlington, VT 05403
(802) 656-2846

Virginia
Don Hardwick, R.R.A. (April)
Health Data Copiers, Inc.
PO Box 2600
Midlothian, VA 23113
(800) 729-5780

Washington
Ann M. Armstrong, R.R.A. (Sept.)
Highline Community Hospital
912 NE 177th Place
Seattle, WA 98155
(206) 548-6176

West Virginia
Beverly A. Tharp, A.R.T. (May)
Route 7, Box 149
Morgantown, WV 26505
(304) 598-1380

Wisconsin
Karen Flood, R.R.A. (April)
2489 Shady Oak Drive
Green Bay, WI 54304
(414) 498-0167

Wyoming

Leta S. Hyde, R.R.A. (May)

811 South 22nd Street

Laramie, WY 82070

(307) 742-2141

Appendix 5
Forms and Form Letters

This appendix contains seven forms and form letters that we have included to help you handle the requests your facility or practice receives. The forms are perforated so they can be easily removed and used, and you are encouraged to photocopy and distribute them throughout your office.

PROCEDURE CHECKLIST FOR RELEASING INFORMATION

Use the following checklist when responding to a request for medical information:

❐ Determine whether or not an authorization was submitted with the request

❐ Check validity of authorization, including:

- ▸ Date (how recent is the consent)

- ▸ Signature (does it match the name on the request; is it the same as on the admission form or initial patient encounter form)

- ▸ The information sought is clearly specified

❐ Verify that the authorization meets federal confidentiality regulations if the patient has a primary diagnosis of drug or alcohol abuse

❐ Request additional information if what is presented does not appear adequate

❐ Post in correspondence log

❐ Notify and obtain the consent of the attending physician, especially regarding requests from patients or if the request indicates any kind of legal action

❐ Locate patient in Patient Index and pull the record

❐ Acknowledge receipt of request

❐ Assemble the material to be sent

❐ Attach redisclosure statement

❐ Have reply checked by supervisor, if applicable

❐ Mail reply

❐ Make a note on the request/authorization and in the log of what was sent, the date sent, and who sent it

❐ File the authorization in the medical record after the request has been processed and the fee collected (if applicable)

This form is adapted, with permission, from information in Helen Marek, *Medicolegal Guidelines and Forms for Hospitals* (Corpus Christi, Tex.: Transcription, Inc., 1979), 47–48.

AUTHORIZATION TO RELEASE INFORMATION

PLEASE PRINT CLEARLY

Patient Name _____
LAST   FIRST   INITIAL

Address _____
STREET   CITY   STATE   ZIP

Phone (_____)_____ Date of Birth _____ Medical Record # _____

I authorize _____ to release medical information from my medical record to:

Name of Doctor, Hospital, etc.: _____

Address: _____

City/State/Zip Code: _____

for the purpose of review/examination and further authorize you to provide such copies thereof as may be requested. The foregoing is subject to such limitation as indicated below:

        ❑ Entire Record
        ❑ Specific Information:
        ❑ Old Records from Previous Physicians

I give special permission to release any information regarding: (initial on line(s) below that you grant us permission to release the information to the above)

_____Substance Abuse   _____Psychiatric/Mental Health Information   _____HIV Information

This authorization will automatically expire one year from the date signed. I understand that I may revoke this consent at any time except to the extent that action has been taken in reliance thereon.

Reason for Request: _____

Signed: _____
(IF NOT PATIENT, STATE RELATIONSHIP)

Witness: _____

FOR OFFICE USE ONLY

Received: _____   Completed by: _____

Completed: _____   Fee Paid:_____

                                      Amount Due/Billed: _____

Disclosure consisted of:_____

_____

_____

NAME:_____

Date: _____

RE: _____

History # / D.O.B.: _____

This is a multiple action form letter with only those items indicated by an "X" being applicable.

IN ANSWER TO YOUR REQUEST FOR MEDICAL INFORMATION

❑ Please see attached medical record copies. NOTE: Request for copies of the entire record will include only the last 2 years of lab work. The attached medical information is CONFIDENTIAL. Subsequent disclosure is not authorized without the specific consent of the patient.

REQUEST FOR ADDITIONAL INFORMATION

❑ Your request is being returned for the following reason(s):

   ❑ We are unable to locate a record of treatment for this individual. Please provide additional information, such as full name of patient at time of treatment, date of birth, history #, or verification of spelling of name. RETURN YOUR REQUEST WITH THE INFORMATION.

   ❑ No record on file for specified dates.

   ❑ Medical information is confidential and can be released only on written consent of patient/patient's legally authorized representative. HAVE THE PATIENT COMPLETE THE ENCLOSED CONSENT AND RETURN YOUR REQUEST WITH THE CONSENT.

   ❑ Authorization date is over 6 months. RETURN YOUR REQUEST WITH A MORE RECENTLY DATED AUTHORIZATION SIGNED BY THE PATIENT/PATIENT'S LEGALLY AUTHORIZED REPRESENTATIVE.

❑ Our charge for releasing records directly to the patient/patient's representative is $_____. If you provide us with the name and address of your new physician, we will send the copies instead, thereby eliminating the charge. Otherwise, make check payable to _____, put patient's name on the check, and return a copy of this letter with check.

❑ Please remit _____, which is our fee for processing your request and photocopying the requested record. Make check payable to_____, reference the patient's name on the check, and return a copy of this letter with check.

❑ Other: _____

_____

_____

_____

_____

_____

FACILITY ABSTRACT FORM

RE:_____

History # / D.O.B.: _____

Date of Admission: _____   Primary Diagnosis: _____

Date of Discharge: _____   Disposition: _____

SIGNIFICANT FINDINGS — HISTORY AND PHYSICAL EXAM

_____
_____
_____
_____

SIGNIFICANT RESULTS — LABORATORY/DIAGNOSTIC PROCEDURES

_____
_____
_____
_____

IMPRESSIONS

_____
_____
_____
_____

TREATMENT PROTOCOL

_____
_____
_____
_____

SURGICAL PROCEDURES AND DATES

_____
_____
_____
_____

PRINCIPAL / DISCHARGE DIAGNOSIS

_____
_____
_____
_____

Authorized Representative _____   Date _____

Note: If you feel it would present a more complete picture of the admission, a discharge summary may accompany or be substituted for the abstract form.

PROVIDER ABSTRACT FORM

RE: _____

Patient #: _____

Date(s) of Patient Care Encounter: _____

Patient Complaint: _____

Primary Diagnosis: _____

SIGNIFICANT FINDINGS — HISTORY AND PHYSICAL EXAM

_____
_____
_____
_____

IMMUNIZATIONS RECORD (FOR CHILDREN)

_____
_____
_____
_____

MEDICATION PROTOCOL

_____
_____
_____
_____

SIGNIFICANT FINDINGS — DIAGNOSTIC / LAB PROCEDURES

_____
_____
_____
_____

SURGICAL PROCEDURES AND DATES

_____
_____
_____

Problem List	Date	Resolution

Principal Diagnoses

_____
_____
_____
_____

Authorized Representative_____Date _____

CONTINUING EDUCATION MODULE

This program has been prior approved by:

The American Health Information Management Association for 10 CE hours.

The Commission on Continuing Education of the New Hampshire Nurses' Association, which is accredited as an approver of continuing education in nursing by the American Nursing Credentialing Center's Commission on Accreditation for 10 Contact Hours.

The following comprehensive review consists of 100 short answer and fill in the blank questions. All answers can be found in *Patient Confidentiality*. Please use the accompanying answer sheets. If more room is needed, use the back of the answer sheets.

Processing fee: $50

Make check or money orders (only) payable to PMIB. U.S. currency only. If you live outside the U.S., please enclose an additional $10

Please mail your completed answer sheets, evaluation, and payment to:

PMIB
2800A Lafayette Road
#203
Portsmouth, NH 03801

The enclosed Certificate of Completion will be returned to you as verification of your successful completion of the activity. Please allow three weeks for delivery. For those having a deadline attached to their continuing education cycle, please postmark your answer sheets *no less* than 30 days prior to the end of your cycle.

Note:

1. Only original answer sheets found in this text will be graded. Photocopies are not acceptable.
2. You may submit a test for grading a maximum of two times under the original processing fee. If you do not pass and are still eligible for regrading, you will be issued "clean" answer sheets as well as your corrected test.

If you know of any association, agency, or facility that would like to sponsor a seminar on "Confidentiality and the Release of Medical Information," please contact PMIB at the above address or call (603) 743-5058.

PLEASE BE ADVISED THAT MEDICODE HAS NEITHER INVOLVEMENT IN NOR RESPONSIBILITY FOR THE AWARDING OF CE CREDITS. DO NOT RETURN YOUR MATERIALS TO MED-INDEX.

SELF-TEST

1. With what medical tradition does ethics regarding the release of medical information originate?

2. Who, historically, has been charged with keeping patients' information confidential?

3. To whom does the physical medical record belong?

4. To whom does the information contained within the medical record belong?

5. For whose benefit is the medical record compiled?

6. Name 5 types of facilities that may engage in the release of information.

   (1)

   (2)

   (3)

   (4)

   (5)

7. List 3 ways by which a request for information can be generated.

   (1)

   (2)

   (3)

8. When deciding what response to make to a request for information, what are the two most important considerations?

   (1)

   (2)

9. Name 4 of the most problematic types of requests.

   (1)

   (2)

   (3)

   (4)

10.   What is of paramount importance when considering release of information issues?

11.   Who are the primary users of medical information?

12. List 4 uses of medical information by secondary users.

   (1)

   (2)

   (3)

   (4)

13. List 5 social users of medical information and their respective uses of the information.

   (1)

   (2)

   (3)

   (4)

   (5)

14. List 4 more than likely improper uses of medical information.

   (1)

   (2)

   (3)

   (4)

15. Who can be held jointly liable for negligence in releasing medical information.?

16. Who is the only person who can authorize the release of information from a record where there is evidence of an abortion having been performed?

17. Who is able to override a minor's refusal (in many states) to release information regarding an abortion if it is in the patient's best physical and mental interests to do so?

18. Define "abstract."

19. Why is the use of abstracts advantageous?

20. Who is required to report cases of probable child abuse?

21. Who, in most states, is encouraged to report voluntarily cases of known child abuse?

22. What information concerning an accident victim may be released to the media unless the patient has specified otherwise?

23. When is an additional information form used?

24. Whose is the final decision as to what information may be released from a facility (except where law or policy dictate otherwise)?

25. Define AIDS/HIV confidential information.

26. What is presently the best safeguard against inadvertently releasing AIDS-related information?

27. What is the American Arbitration Association?

28. Through whom should requests from the facility's attorney or insurer be channeled?

29. Who, in order of priority, is able to authorize the release of information from a medical record?

   (1)

   (2)

   (3)

   (4)

30. List the 9 ingredients of a valid authorization.

   (1)

   (2)

   (3)

   (4)

   (5)

   (6)

   (7)

   (8)

   (9)

31. What 2 clauses should be added to a general authorization as safeguards?

   (1)

   (2)

32. Under what circumstances are minors the only ones legally authorized to consent to the release of information from their respective records?

33. When are letters of testamentary issued?

34. What are letters of administration?

35. List in order of priority, the persons that may authorize the release of information from a deceased person's record in the event a legal representative has not been named.

   (1)

   (2)

   (3)

   (4)

   (5)

36. Whose consent should be obtained prior to releasing any information concerning the birth of a baby?

37. How should copies of birth certificates be retained by a hospital?

38. A _____ _____ may be set for copying information from the record, for the completion of abstracts, and for record searches.

39. Medical staff committee reports compiled for the purpose of evaluating the quality of care are _____ or _____ and as such are not admissible as _____ in any court action.

40. List 4 examples of contracted services.

   (1)

   (2)

   (3)

   (4)

41. With one exception, what is the one request for a medical record that cannot be refused?

42. Unlike news of a birth, news of a death is _____ _____.

43. List 5 diseases whose occurrence a physician may be responsible for reporting.

   (1)

   (2)

   (3)

   (4)

   (5)

44. Persons representing the armed forces or draft board (Selective Service) who wish to review a medical record must present _____ _____ and must _____ and _____ the patient's authorization.

45. Federal rules applying to drug and alcohol abuse records are found in what government publication?

46. What facilities are affected by the federal protection of drug and alcohol abuse records?

   (1)

   (2)

   (3)

   (4)

47. Drug and alcohol abuse records of those in the military fall under the jurisdiction of the _____ _____ ____ _____ _____ . Any exchange of information must occur exclusively between the various _____ of the armed forces or between the _____ _____ and the _____ _____.

48. In the absence of a valid authorization, federally protected drug and alcohol abuse records may only be disclosed pursuant to a _____ _____ and then only if a _____ is held and the record of that _____ indicates good cause exists for the disclosure.

49. A valid authorization for the release of drug and alcohol abuse records (federally protected) must contain what 9 ingredients?

 (1)

 (2)

 (3)

 (4)

 (5)

 (6)

 (7)

 (8)

 (9)

50. A patient's _____/_____ to an inpatient facility for drug or alcohol abuse treatment can only be acknowledged to visitors/callers with the patient's _____ _____ .

51. Except in those states that allow drug and alcohol abuse treatment for minors without parental consent, the consent of both the _____ and the _____ or _____ is required for the release of information.

52. A statement on Prohibition on _____ must accompany any written disclosure from a drug or alcohol abuse patient's record.

53. Define "emancipated minor."

54. When a patient is being transferred to an extended care facility, what should the transferring facility's report include?

55. When is the only time medical information should be released and transmitted by fax?

56. Documents faxed on _____ _____ should be copied prior to being filed in the medical record as _____ _____ tends to deteriorate over time.

57. List 7 government agencies that have the power to subpoena medical records.

 (1)

 (2)

 (3)

 (4)

 (5)

 (6)

 (7)

58. List 4 ways in which the medical record is used as an impersonal document.

    (1)

    (2)

    (3)

    (4)

59. It is generally accepted that by initiating a malpractice suit, the patient waives the _____ ___ _____ of the pertinent medical information.

60. What are the 2 reasons for maintaining a correspondence and/or release of information log?

    (1)

    (2)

61. What information should be contained in the log?

62. In case of malpractice, the record in question should be reviewed for _____ , _____ ___ _____ , _____ and _____ of _____ and checked for _____ and _____ .

63. The rules governing Medicaid call for the _____ disclosure of medical information by a provider or facility specifically for the purpose of _____ _____ .

64. _____ is much like Medicaid in that routine disclosure of information pertinent to processing claims is a condition of coverage.

65. In what 5 situations would nursing home resident abuse reporting be required?

    (1)

    (2)

    (3)

    (4)

    (5)

66. Most states, in keeping with the general trend toward _____ _____ allow the patients to have free access to their medical records.

67. The _____ _____ , which prevails in federal institutions, gives patients access to their records and allows them to _____ and/or _____ them.

68. If a physician makes a determination that access to the record would not be in the best interests of the patient, a notation of that determination should be made _____ _____ _____ .

69. What 4 things should be considered when deciding whether or not the patient should have access to the record?

   (1)

   (2)

   (3)

   (4)

70. Persons receiving photocopies of records should be reminded in writing that the information is to

   (1)

   (2)

71. A _____ physician may only have access to the records of those patients he or she is currently treating. This is being more strictly enforced at present.

72. At the request of a _____ physician, an abstract of medical information may be sent to a _____ physician who is not a member of the medical staff without the patient's consent.

73. One or more persons within a facility should be specifically designated to handle all requests from the _____ .

74. A hospital _____ _____ that a public figure is hospitalized unless confirmation has been forbidden by the patient or the physician or the patient is hospitalized for substance or alcohol abuse at a facility whose records are protected by federal law.

75. Any inquiries concerning a rape victim should be referred to the _____ .

76. Information pertaining to a rape should only be released to _____ _____ _____ if the victim has implied consent by deciding to press charges.

77. Any facility or provider, when responding to a request for information, should attach a _____ _____ to the information so the receiving party will not in turn release that information to a third party.

78. Give 5 examples of when a refusal to honor a request for information would be in order.

   (1)

   (2)

   (3)

   (4)

   (5)

79. A _____ for the _____ of _____ is an increasingly popular method by which attorneys pursuing the discovery process in a lawsuit obtain pertinent medical information.

80. List 5 conditions/incidents whose occurrence a knowledgeable and responsible person may be required to report.

   (1)

   (2)

   (3)

   (4)

   (5)

81. The results of research studies should not be published without the permission of the _____ _____ .

82. For the purposes of research, information from medical records may be utilized without the _____ _____ .

83. Policies for the release of information to outside researchers should be established by the _____ _____ and _____ _____ .

84. Records should be reviewed by interested individuals in the presence of either _____ _____ _____ or the _____ _____ for the case.

85. The hospital _____ _____ _____ on which a patient is hospitalized is confidential information.

86. A request by a student of an allied health program to review a patient's record after the patient has been discharged may require the authorization of the _____ _____ .

87. Upon being served with a subpoena, immediately inquire as to

   (1)

   (2)

88. A Subpoena Duces Tecum is more properly known as a _____ _____ ____ _____ ____ _____ _____ .

89. When assembling medical information in response to a subpoena, check the state statute to see if _____ _____ , _____ , _____ _____ _____ , and copies of _____ and _____ _____ remain or are removed from the record.

90. Any discrepancies found when reviewing a record for completeness and integrity prior to responding to a subpoena should be brought to the attention of the _____ _____ and _____ _____ .

91. As a witness in court, one testifies that the medical record was created in the _____ _____ of _____ .

92. A medical record is never left when answering a _____ subpoena for discovery purposes.

93. Inquiries from the media concerning suicides or attempted suicides should be referred to the _____ .

94. Ideally, telephone requests for medical information should only be honored in _____ _____ _____ situations.

95. Telephone requests should always be handled via a _____ _____ procedure.

96. For what type of treatments can a patient be temporarily transferred to another facility?

97. True or False: A minor who has been treated for venereal disease is the only one authorized to release information pertaining to that treatment.

98. List 3 situations where voluntary disclosures are encouraged by most state statutes.

   (1)

   (2)

   (3)

99. Workers Compensation is administered within each individual _____ .

100. Any individual eligible for and who applies for Workers Compensation automatically authorizes the release of information specifically pertaining to the _____ _____ _____ _____ .

CERTIFICATE OF CE COMPLETION

◆

Activity: Self-test for Patient Confidentiality: An Alphabetized Guide to the Release of Medical Information

This activity has been prior approved by:

The American Health Information Management Association for 10 CE hours

The Commission on Continuing Education of the New Hampshire Nurses' Association, which is accredited as an approver of continuing education in nursing by the American Nursing Credentialing Center's Commission on Accreditation for 10 contact hours

Name _____

Credentials _____

Address _____

City _____

State _____

Zip _____

Professional Association _____

◆ ◆ ◆

For Office Use Only

Score _____

Date _____

Hours _____

_____

Signature / Authorized Program Representative

INDEPENDENT STUDY EVALUATION

Activity: Self-test for Confidentiality and the Release of Medical Information

Dear Participant:

I hope you enjoyed this activity and found it informative. Your feedback is necessary and appreciated. Please read the following statements and then circle the numbers that you feel best apply.

1 — Poor   2 — Fair   3 — Good   4 — Excellent   5 — Outstanding

1. Relevance of content to subject: Confidentiality and the release of medical information	1 2 3 4 5
2. Clarity of content	1 2 3 4 5

3. The activity was successful in helping the participant be able to:

a.	explain patient confidentiality's origin in ethics, ownership of medical records, legal implications of breaching confidentiality, and the process of releasing information as a profit center	1 2 3 4 5
b.	discuss the numerous users of information	1 2 3 4 5
c.	define the uses of information	1 2 3 4 5
d.	identify problematic types of requests	1 2 3 4 5
e.	discuss the many factors that relate to patient confidentiality	1 2 3 4 5
f.	formulate a confidentiality policy that protects the patients' right to privacy and the interests of the organization	1 2 3 4 5
g.	describe the process by which information is released	1 2 3 4 5

4. Effectiveness of the self-test module as a learning tool	1 2 3 4 5

5. Do you feel the knowledge obtained will be useful in your particular work setting?

6. Would you recommend this activity to a co-worker or friend?

7. What did you like best about the self-test module?

8. What was the most important thing you learned and will remember?

9. How many hours did it take you to complete the activity?

Comments/suggestions:

Name_____